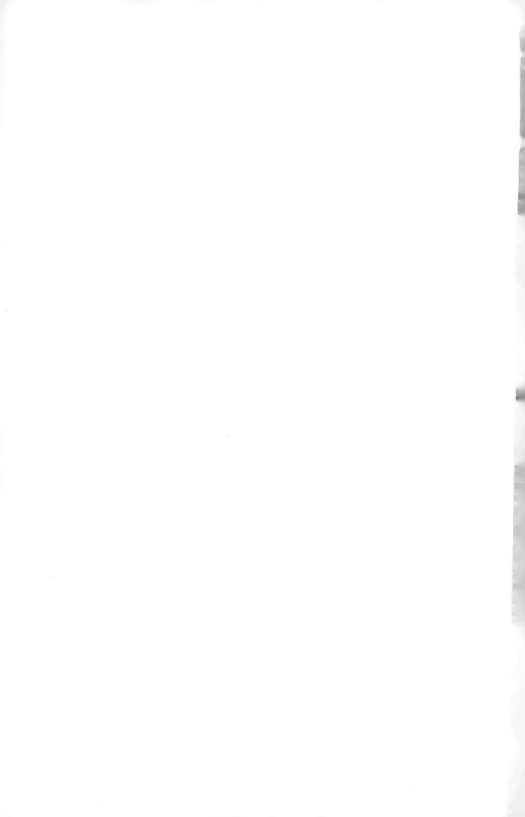

THE PAIN EPIDEMIC

THE PAIN EPIDEMIC

A Guide to Issues, Symptoms, Treatments, and Wellness

Don Goldenberg

ROWMAN & LITTLEFIELD
Lanham • Boulder • New York • London

This book represents reference material only. It is not intended as a medical manual, and the data presented here are meant to assist the reader in making informed choices regarding wellness. This book is not a replacement for treatment(s) that the reader's personal physician may have suggested. If the reader believes he or she is experiencing a medical issue, professional medical help is recommended. Mention of particular products, companies, or authorities in this book does not entail endorsement by the publisher or author.

Published by Rowman & Littlefield
An imprint of The Rowman & Littlefield Publishing Group, Inc.
4501 Forbes Boulevard, Suite 200, Lanham, Maryland 20706
https://rowman.com

6 Tinworth Street, London SE11 5AL, United Kingdom

British Library Cataloguing in Publication Information Available

Library of Congress Cataloging-in-Publication Data
Names: Goldenberg, Don L., author.
Title: The pain epidemic : a guide to issues, symptoms, treatments, and
    wellness / Don Goldenberg.
Description: Lanham : Rowman & Littlefield, [2020] | Includes biblio-
    graphical references and index.
Identifiers: LCCN 2020009908 (print) | LCCN 2020009909 (ebook) |
    ISBN 9781538138359 (hardcover) | ISBN 9781538138366 (epub)
Subjects: LCSH: Chronic pain. | Chronic pain—Treatment.
Classification: LCC RB127 .G653 2020 (print) | LCC RB127 (ebook) |
    DDC 616/.0472—dc23
LC record available at https://lccn.loc.gov/2020009908
LC ebook record available at https://lccn.loc.gov/2020009909

CONTENTS

INTRODUCTION

My personal odyssey to better understand and treat chronic pain began forty years ago. My wife, Patty, an excellent athlete and tennis player, was struck in the left eye with a tennis ball. She could not see through the blood that pooled in the outer chamber of her eye, and we worried that she might lose sight in that eye. Her treatment consisted of two weeks of complete bed rest with a patch over the injured eye. Fortunately, the eye healed and her sight was restored. However, it quickly became apparent that she was having difficulty recovering her normal health.

Patty began suffering from generalized muscle pain and exhaustion. During the two weeks of bed rest, as frequently happens to people in that situation, Patty had difficulty distinguishing day from night, and her sleep became very erratic. However, the insomnia persisted for Patty; she began waking up frequently during the night and had difficulty getting back to sleep. She described waking up feeling like "a truck just ran me over." Muscle soreness and exhaustion prevented her from getting back to her regular exercise routine. Her neck and back pain were constant and accompanied by severe headaches.

In addition, she began complaining of a number of seemingly unrelated new symptoms. These included abdominal discomfort and cramping with bouts of constipation and diarrhea. Patty also experienced urinary frequency and urgency, often accompanied by bladder and pelvic discomfort.

As a rheumatologist, my first thought was that Patty had developed a connective tissue disease such as rheumatoid arthritis or systemic lupus erythematosus (lupus). These are diseases that occur most often in young women, and they often present with generalized pain and fatigue. However, when I examined her, there was no swelling around her joints, the cardinal finding in systemic arthritis. Neither was there any obvious weakness or neurologic abnormality. What I did find was a lot of tenderness almost anywhere that I probed her muscles and joints. Following the unwritten medical rule of never treating your family, I decided to send Patty to one of the more prominent rheumatologists in Boston for an expert consultation.

He ordered numerous blood tests and X-rays and told me that he also was concerned that Patty might have an immune disease, such as lupus or scleroderma. One of the laboratory tests, the antinuclear antibody, a marker for lupus, was positive. However, that test can be positive in healthy women, and all her other blood tests were normal. He treated Patty with a short course of prednisone, a corticosteroid that often works wonders in systemic rheumatic diseases. The prednisone did not help her symptoms but made her sleep disturbances much worse, which aggravated her exhaustion.

We then began a yearlong search for answers and consulted with a number of different medical specialists. A neurologist whom I greatly admired felt that Patty probably had a neuropathy. Patty underwent painful nerve conduction velocity tests to her arms and legs. The results were equivocal. A brief trial with a medication used to treat neuropathy was not helpful. We saw a new general internist, who ran a battery of blood tests and X-rays but again without finding any clues to her symptoms.

As the year dragged on, Patty and I both suspected that some of her symptoms could be related to depression. Usually cheerful and upbeat, Patty said, "This is really getting to me." She had no previous bouts of depression, although both her mother and sister had a history of mood disorders. Patty had worked in my office for years, and we were both keenly aware of the intricate relationship between depression and pain and fatigue.

Just then I read a medical report on fibromyalgia. I had heard of fibromyalgia, which had also been termed "fibrositis," but my rheumatology mentors had dismissed it as a wastebasket term for poorly understood aches and pains. However, this new article on fibromyalgia described every one of Patty's symptoms to a tee. It was as if I was reading her yearlong medical history. Fibromyalgia patients were most commonly women, between ages thirty and fifty. They all had unexplained generalized muscle pain and exhaustion with no evidence for a systemic inflammatory or immune disease. The article also reported that there were specific locations in the body where patients with fibromyalgia were most tender to palpation when modest pressure was applied. I proceeded to search for these on Patty and she had all of these "tender points."

Over the next few days, I read every article on fibromyalgia that I could find. Patty's gastrointestinal symptoms were consistent with irritable bowel syndrome, and the urinary frequency and urgency were typical of chronic pelvic and bladder pain syndrome, both present in the majority of women with fibromyalgia. Most patients with fibromyalgia also suffered from sleep and mood disturbances and chronic headaches, as did Patty. One medical report suggested that treatment with a small amount of amitriptyline was helpful for the sleep problems and might decrease the pain of fibromyalgia. So I prescribed a tiny amount (10 mg) of amitriptyline.

After just a few days, Patty's sleep improved, and her exhaustion began to subside. Within the next few weeks, most of her muscle soreness and generalized achiness also improved. She was able to start walking outside and rejoined some of her exercise classes. Over the next year, almost all her symptoms subsided and she was back to her outgoing, enthusiastic self. Patty continued to take between 20 and 30 mg of amitriptyline at bedtime, and with that small dose, her sleep was generally quite good, especially if she sustained her exercise routine.

I became more and more interested in fibromyalgia and began to diagnose it frequently in my own patients. Looking back, I recognized that I had missed that diagnosis in many patients over the previous decade. Like most rheumatologists, I had been trained to search for a rheumatic disease, such as rheumatoid arthritis or lupus. After eliminating those possibilities, I would tell patients that they needn't worry about a serious immune disorder. However, I was unable to give them a specific diagnosis or advise them about a therapeutic program.

It became apparent that there was a lot of research to be done to better understand and treat fibromyalgia, and I became determined to play a major role in that endeavor. Over the next few years, I joined with a number of rheumatologists to direct clinical and basic research about fibromyalgia and became an internationally recognized authority on this condition.

One of my many questions about fibromyalgia was related to the mind-body interface that seemed to me so important in driving the condition. My first research article was devoted to evaluating clinical and biologic markers of depression in patients with fibromyalgia. The results demonstrated that fibromyalgia, in contrast to what many "experts" thought, was not simply a manifestation of depression. However, we did find evidence for increased mood disturbances in patients and family members with fibromyalgia compared to the general population.

I had always been intrigued by the complex interplay of our emotions and our mood with physical symptoms. Initially I had wanted to be a psychiatrist or psychologist, but somewhere along the way my career veered into rheumatology. Rheumatologists deal with chronic diseases, and I embraced the long-standing relationship I had with my patients. I was able to get to know them as people rather than just as patients.

Personal experience is always our best teacher. Certainly, Patty's illness was the driving force behind my forty-year undertaking to better understand and treat fibromyalgia. It resulted in my establishing the Arthritis/Fibromyalgia Clinic at the Newton-Wellesley Hospital in Massachusetts and eventually evaluating twenty thousand fibromyalgia patients. I was invited to speak all over the world and was interviewed for the *New York Times*, the *Boston Globe*, and on *Today* and *Good Morning America*.

Another factor that spurred my personal commitment to better comprehend chronic pain and suffering was my own medical problems, which began ten years after those of my wife. I, too, had had bouts of unexplained exhaustion since my early thirties. These were often attributed to a flu and sometimes treated with antibiotics. In addition, I suffered from monthly migraine headaches. Constantly trying to determine what triggered the migraine attacks, I kept experimenting with my diet, drinking less coffee, and trying various supplements, all to no avail.

Suddenly, in 1993, the headaches became daily and much more severe. As had Patty, I consulted various subspecialists, including my internist; an ophthalmologist; an allergist; an ear, nose, and throat specialist; and a neurologist. The neurologist ordered brain magnetic resonance imaging (MRI), which revealed a small abnormality in the right side of my brain. No one could be certain whether this was the cause of my headaches, but a neurosurgeon recommended that it be removed because of the possibility of a brain tumor. Needless to say, my whole life flashed through my mind, and I imagined the worst.

The surgery went as planned, and the lesion was successfully removed. However, when back in the intensive care unit, I had a grand mal seizure, witnessed by Patty. Over the ensuing forty-eight hours, I had two more seizures, which fortunately I have no memory of. Eventually I was discharged from the hospital and put on an antiseizure medication, which made me feel quite exhausted. We received good news that the brain lesion was not malignant, and my fear of dying from brain cancer disappeared. However, because of the recent seizure and the new medication, I could not drive or work for a while and had difficulty concentrating. After getting back to work, I was not feeling like myself, just as Patty had described herself. I was exhausted all the time and simple activities became a struggle. I was having difficulty getting to sleep, usually because my mind was racing with thoughts like,

Will I have another seizure? What is the matter with me? When will I start feeling better? Is this all in my head?

This personal experience, as well as those of Patty, has heightened my awareness of the adverse impact of medical uncertainty. We all want an answer as to the cause of our medical symptoms. How else will we get better? I was no different, obsessing over what was being missed or wondering what would soon happen to me. When would the other shoe fall?

I did recognize that my insomnia and exhaustion likely were tied in with my worsening mood and my frustration with the lack of any answers. My internist referred me to a psychiatrist, who confirmed that I was depressed. He put me on a low dose of an antidepressant, and I began weekly counseling. I felt much better within a few weeks and was back to baseline after a few months.

Patty's and my struggle with these intertwined physical and psychological symptoms motivated me to dedicate much of my career to better understanding and treating fibromyalgia and related chronic pain disorders. In more recent years, I have focused on providing better medical information to patients and families dealing with chronic pain and authored two books, *Chronic Illness and Uncertainty* and *Fibromyalgia*.

The Pain Epidemic broadens this discussion and provides new, critical insight into the most important aspects of understanding chronic pain. The first part of the book focuses on key issues, including the size and impact of our current pain epidemic. A biopsychological model of chronic pain will be described in order to explain the genetic, environmental, and gender underpinnings of chronic pain. The paucity of credible information on chronic pain, both for health-care professionals and the public, is discussed and suggestions made to search out reputable sources.

The next portion of the book discusses the most common chronic pain conditions, including fibromyalgia, chronic low back and neck pain, and migraine and other chronic headaches. The symptoms and diagnosis of each of these conditions, including their common nature, will be reviewed. Case histories of famous subjects as well as my own patients will better illustrate these conditions.

Understanding the shared nature of these chronic pain conditions helps the reader accept the universal principles of pain management discussed in the final part of the book. This begins with medications used to treat chronic pain, including a chapter on the pitfalls of opioids and the promise of cannabis-related products. Nonpharmacologic pain management is then detailed, including exercise, yoga, tai chi, and mind-body techniques, such as cognitive behavioral therapy and meditation. Successful chronic pain management requires an interdisciplinary health-care team, and I suggest ways to organize that. Finally, echoing what a number of my patients have taught me, I provide specific recommendations to better understand and treat your chronic pain.

1

CHRONIC PAIN

A Public Health Epidemic

I first met Virginia when she was fifty-eight and was referred to me regarding her lifelong history of chronic pain. She described herself as having been a sickly child and having suffered from severe menstrual cramps and headaches as a teenager. Often Virginia would wake up feeling "sore and achy all over, like I had the flu." After the birth of her only child, Virginia began to experience severe pelvic pain and bladder irritability. Extensive laboratory and radiologic testing was unrevealing. The bladder and pelvic pain was treated with topical medications and chemicals instilled in her bladder, none of which helped. During the ten years prior to our meeting, Virginia was in constant pain, always involving her neck and back but sometimes including her extremities. She described the pain as "deep, in my muscles," but at times it had a burning quality. Virginia's medical history was strikingly similar to Patty's.

One out of every three Americans live with chronic pain, usually defined as lasting for at least three to six months.[1] Pain is the number one reason we seek medical care, and chronic pain accounts for 40 percent of all doctor visits. The yearly cost of chronic pain in the United States is between $560 billion and $630 billion, higher than that of heart disease, diabetes, and cancer combined.[2] Low back pain, neck pain, and headaches are the leading causes of disability in the United States.[3] Annually, a person with chronic pain generates about $5,000 greater health-care costs than one without chronic pain.

Chronic pain increases with advancing age. As our population lives longer, a growing number of Americans suffer from chronic pain. Up to 50 percent of older Americans live in chronic pain. The rise of obesity also has increased the prevalence of chronic pain. Certain populations are more prone to chronic pain. All types of chronic pain are more common in women. It is present in up to 50 percent of military veterans and is more common among Hispanics and African Americans.

The prevalence of chronic pain correlates with low income and less education. A person with no high school diploma is 1.3 times more likely to have severe headaches or migraine than a person with some college education.[4] Low back pain is present in 35 percent of the population below the poverty level, compared to 24 percent above the poverty level.[5]

Chronic pain is the most common cause of work loss worldwide. Loss of mobility in daily activities results in a vicious cycle that leads to unemployment and disability. A study of the US workforce found that individuals with chronic pain missed an average of five to six more workdays per year than did people with no pain.[6] This factored out to twelve billion hours of productive work time lost, with an estimated $220 billion in lost wages yearly in the United States.

Chronic pain decreases quality of life, interfering with physical function as well as with our emotional and social well-being. Chronic pain promotes depression and often results in social isolation. These effects begin early in life, as noted in a study of fifteen thousand adolescents, one-third of whom had chronic pain.[7] Those with chronic pain had lower academic achievement, poor vocational function, earlier parenthood, and lower adult income levels.

Chronic pain shortens life expectancy, due in part to the association of pain with depression. There is a twofold increased risk of suicide in every chronic pain disorder. This has been well documented in patients with fibromyalgia, chronic low back pain, and migraine.[8] Suicide risk increases with the duration and severity of pain and correlates with levels of insomnia, depression, and helplessness. The increased mortality in people with chronic pain is also linked to decreased mobility and being more sedentary. These are associated with less exercise and subsequent increased risk of obesity, diabetes, and cardiovascular disease.

Although chronic pain has long been recognized as a major health problem, its prevalence has been increasing. For example, there has been an 800 percent increase in hospital admissions for chronic pain during the past twenty years.[9] There are many reasons for this increased incidence of chronic pain, including the aging of the population and the increased burden of all age-related, chronic disorders. Multiple studies have also demonstrated a correlation of the rise in obesity with the increase in a number of painful disorders, such as osteoarthritis of the hips and knees. Obesity increases the load and strain on weight-bearing joints, including the hips and knees.

The increased prevalence of chronic pain disorders like low back pain, fibromyalgia, and migraine is not so easily explained, since each of these conditions is common in younger adults and has little to do with body weight or trauma. A study of chronic low back pain conducted in North Carolina found "an alarming increase in the prevalence of chronic low back pain from 1992 to 2006 . . . across all population subgroups."[10] The prevalence of chronic low back pain more than doubled over the period, from about 4 percent to more than 10 percent. For women of all ages and men ages forty-five to fifty-four, the prevalence of chronic low back pain nearly tripled. Health-care spending in the United States for low back pain increased from $8 billion to $18 billion from 1990 to 2000.[11]

The miracles of modern-day medicine have wiped out many lethal diseases and have allowed patients with cancer, heart disease, diabetes, and autoimmune diseases to live longer and more productively. There have been no similar advances in the treatment of chronic pain. Much of this failure can be traced to centuries-old medical misconceptions about pain.

Physicians have been taught that medical conditions were either physical or mental disorders. In 1641 the French philosopher Rene Descartes, in *Meditations on First Philosophy*, suggested that the mind and body were separate, although closely aligned.[12] During the next few centuries, diseases were defined by body system pathology. Doctors were trained in a biomedical disease model, wherein disease must be diagnosed objectively, with tissue biopsy and notation of laboratory or radiologic abnormalities. Physicians were taught that medical conditions were either physical or mental disorders.

Pain, according to Cartesian philosophy, was a physical sensation transmitted as a noxious signal to a specific brain region. Following the biomedical disease model, chronic pain was classified by its organ source. Inflammatory pain, such as from rheumatoid arthritis, was caused by joint inflammation causing structural deterioration. Neuropathic pain, as from diabetic neuropathy, was caused by peripheral nerve damage. The degree of physical damage was considered to be proportional to the pain severity. Accordingly, pain would be restricted to the site of injury or damage. It was assumed that pain would vanish once the tissue healed or the damage was fixed, such as by replacing an arthritic joint.

Pain management has been directed at curing the disease or fixing the injury. Little research has been devoted to chronic pain itself, and very few physicians have made it a career. Those who did have focused on the potential structural causes of pain. Physicians and patients readily understand that the degree of nerve or joint damage should reflect the severity of one's pain. But what do we conclude when there is no obvious joint or nerve damage?

Pain is our warning sign that something is wrong. In its acute form, pain is our friend and essential to our survival. The response to acute pain is immediate, requires no conscious thought, and is easy to understand. When we touch something hot, our hand immediately withdraws. The speed of that withdraw reaction is proportional to the severity of the painful stimulus. However, when pain persists, it quickly becomes our foe, not our friend. Rather than being protective, chronic pain leads to misery and suffering.

For centuries, pain was seen as a purely physical state, like temperature, blood pressure, heart rate, and breathing. This implied that pain could be graded objectively. In the 1990s pain was earmarked as the "fifth vital sign." Medical personnel checkmarked happy to very sad faces daily in hospital records. This raised health-care providers' awareness—and that of the public in general—of the importance of pain, but it was misleading. There are no pain tests analogous to taking our temperature or blood pressure. This narrow biomedical model of chronic pain failed to account for the subjective and very personal nature of pain. Chronic pain is a biopsychological condition, yet health care continued to focus on its biomedical aspects.

A biopsychological illness model rejects mind-body dualism. Chronic pain no longer would be boxed into neat categories such as peripheral (structural or inflammatory) and central. It became increasingly apparent that the central nervous system, via pain mechanisms, emotions, and cognition, modified every type of pain, no matter the initial source. In 1994 a new definition of pain was agreed upon: "An unpleasant sensory and emotional experience associated with actual or potential tissue damage, or described in terms of such damage. . . . Pain is always subjective. . . . It is unquestionably a sensation in a part or parts of the body, but it is also always unpleasant and therefore also an emotional experience."[13]

Chronic pain may be present without any obvious structural damage. In my own field of rheumatology, the most striking example is fibromyalgia, where years of searching for muscle or joint damage had proved futile. I authored a counterpoint to a medical article written by a prominent rheumatologist proclaiming that fibromyalgia was "not real, in contrast to legitimate diseases, like rheumatoid arthritis,"[14] the message being that all real diseases must have an acknowledged physical source of chronic pain.

The most extraordinary example of pain persisting in the absence of bodily damage is phantom limb syndrome, initially described by a French surgeon, Ambroise Paré, in the sixteenth century.[15] Between 50 to 80 percent of amputees report chronic pain and other unpleasant sensations at the site of the amputated limb. It feels as if the amputated limb is still there, crying out in misery. Following the biomedical disease model, these sensations were thought to be related to irritated sensory nerves at the amputated stump. That theory was debunked after a century of misguided treatments. Phantom limb pain is now known to be driven by changes in the central nervous system.[16] Phantom limb pain arises outside the body's physical border, but the brain connection to the severed limb remains spatially intact.

Even in diseases with obvious organ damage or dysfunction, the severity of pain varies greatly from one person to the next. For example, in osteoarthritis some patients with severely destroyed knees on X-ray have little pain whereas others with minimal damage report severe pain. Pain experts coined the term "central pain" or "central sensitization" to denote pain arising solely from the central nervous system, requiring no peripheral (bodily) input.

Central pain was initially considered to be dysfunctional. If there was no peripheral (body) damage (danger), there should be no activation of our intrinsic warning system. Placing pain in a biomedical disease model also suggested that structural, inflammatory, and neuropathic pain were physical diseases whereas central pain was primarily a mental disorder. Central pain was "all in your head" and considered to be an exaggerated, aberrant emotional response. Chronic pain conditions, such as fibromyalgia, were classified as psychosomatic. Patients with a central pain disorder, like fibromyalgia or chronic headaches, were often stigmatized as constitutionally weak or as exaggerating their symptoms for attention or to obtain drugs.

We now recognize that chronic pain is a disease in itself. During the past fifty years, conditions like fibromyalgia, migraine, chronic low back pain, and irritable bowel syndrome have been more readily diagnosed and better understood within a biopsychological illness framework. This model recognizes that chronic pain involves a complex interplay of genetic, biologic, and personal factors, unique to every individual. Pain no longer can be thought of as a purely physical sensation.

In 2011 the prestigious Institute of Medicine published the important document, *Relieving Pain in America: A Blueprint for Transforming Prevention, Care, Education and Research*.[17] One of the charges for the Institute of Medicine's committee was to "increase the recognition of pain as a significant health problem in the United States." Important conclusions from that report included these statements: "Chronic pain is the result of biological, psychological and social factors, has distinct pathology and can be a disease in itself. . . . It is important to prevent the transition from the acute to the chronic state of pain through early intervention. . . . Public health pain education can help counter the myths, misunderstandings, stereotypes, and stigma that hinder better care."

In 2019 the International Classification of Diseases, eleventh revision (ICD-11), established a diagnostic coding system for chronic pain.[18] For the first time, chronic pain or "chronic primary pain," was recognized as a disease in and of itself. With this recognition comes the realization that we are mired in a pain epidemic. Chronic pain is pervasive, costly, poorly understood, and inadequately treated. The hundreds of billions of wasted dollars spent on costly, invasive procedures and on chronic opioids have only added to our advancing wave of chronic pain. The Institute of Medicine concluded that "effective pain management is a moral imperative, a professional responsibility and the duty of people in the healing professions."

IMPORTANT POINTS ABOUT THE CHRONIC PAIN EPIDEMIC

- We are currently in an epidemic of chronic pain.

- Chronic pain is more common in women and certain ethnic groups, and it increases with age and with lower income and education levels.
- Chronic pain interferes with every aspect of our lives.
- Chronic pain shortens life expectancy.
- Chronic pain must be recognized as a disease in itself.

2

MIND *AND/*OR BODY

Janet was sent to me by one of our staff psychiatrists. The psychiatrist had been seeing her on and off for a number of years after she developed postpartum depression when she was twenty-nine. Since then Janet had dealt with bouts of anxiety and was successfully treated with counseling. At age thirty-six Janet began having difficulty sleeping, followed by feelings of exhaustion, difficulty concentrating, and generalized pain that was especially prominent in her neck and arms. Janet recalled having similar pain when she was diagnosed with postpartum depression. She was concerned that these new symptoms were signals that her depression was returning. Janet, like Patty and me, were worried that maybe "it is all in my head." This is an unfortunate result of the obsolete notion that pain is either physical or mental.

Emotional and cognitive factors impact every chronic disease, including heart disease and diabetes. However, in chronic pain the absence of objective physical measures can make it easy to conclude that the pain is purely psychological. Physicians must rely on patients' self-reporting to quantify pain severity. Furthermore, since every human being experiences pain at times, those with chronic pain may be considered constitutionally weak or simply unable to cope.

By definition, chronic pain is a condition in which pain persists beyond the normal healing process. It cannot be explained simply by injury or organ disease. Chronic pain is primarily a central nervous system disorder, driven by the brain reorganizing itself, referred to as "neuroplasticity." When pain persists, it becomes hardwired, leaving behind a blueprint that remodels the brain and spinal cord. Our pain gauge is amped up. This plays out clinically with generalized body pain and irritability.

Fibromyalgia patients have often been likened to the young maiden in Hans Christian Andersen's fairy tale "The Princess and the Pea."[1] Her sensitive nature was tested by placing a pea in her bed underneath huge mattresses and twenty featherbeds. Despite all the cushioning, the next morning she told the prince that she couldn't sleep because something hard in her bed had bruised her. The prince treasured her super awareness, crowning her his princess. However, most medical professionals find such hypersensitivity aberrant and unworthy of validation.

This brain-derived hyperreactivity, termed "central sensitization," is characteristic of most chronic pain disorders.[2] Central sensitization also accounts for the excess sensitivity to noise, odors, foods, and other environmental stimuli in conditions such as fibromyalgia, migraine, and irritable bowel syndrome. It may make chronic pain patients unable to tolerate medications. Until recently there were no ways to observe and document this neuroplasticity. It was easy to conclude that such hypersensitivity was a character flaw.

Brain imaging, such as magnetic resonance imaging (MRI), has provided a window to document the functional and structural brain reprocessing that results from chronic pain. This involves a series of biologic events that can restructure the pain matrix of the brain. Certain brain chemicals, such as glutamate and dopamine, are activated, and their levels correlate with pain severity and duration.[3] Loss of brain gray matter has been noted in a number of chronic pain conditions, and such structural shifts are proportional to the degree and duration of pain. These physical changes are present in brain regions that transmit pain, such as the insula, the prefrontal cortex, the thalamus, and the amygdala. If the chronic pain is alleviated, such structural changes often normalize.

In chronic pain the connectivity of various brain regions that transmit pain signals is transformed. The insula is the brain region most responsible for pain perception. The anterior insula is involved in the cognitive and affective dimension of pain, while the mid and posterior insula direct the sensory aspects of pain. Functional MRI (fMRI) has demonstrated that in chronic pain there are changes in how the insula communicates with other pain-processing brain regions. A neuroimaging map of chronic pain rewiring can now be drawn.[4] Neural signatures have already been proposed for the diagnosis of chronic pain conditions, such as fibromyalgia, although this approach is not yet ready for prime-time applicability.[5]

A biopsychological illness model explains the near-universal association of depression, fatigue, and sleep disturbances with chronic pain. Depression is present in the vast majority of patients with chronic pain and has been extensively written about as the pain/depression dyad.[6] A lifetime history of depression is present in 10 percent of the general population but in 70 percent of patients with chronic pain.[7] The association of mood disturbances with pain is bidirectional: greater pain equals greater depression; more depression leads to greater pain severity. This correlation of mood disturbances with pain is not only true in conditions such as fibromyalgia and migraine but also in rheumatic diseases, including rheumatoid arthritis or osteoarthritis.

Chronic pain and depression result in nearly identical central nervous system remodeling. Neurotransmitters, including serotonin, dopamine, and norepinephrine are decreased in patients with chronic pain and with depression. Brain imaging in patients with depression and in those with chronic pain reveals similar structural and functional changes in the prefrontal cortex, the hippocampus, and the amygdala.

Exhaustion and sleep disturbances are present in 60 percent to 90 percent of patients with chronic pain.[8] Poor sleep is one of the strongest predictors of developing chronic, widespread pain.[9]

Chronic pain is most often associated with disturbances in deep, stage 4 sleep, termed "restorative sleep." Primary sleep disturbances, including sleep apnea and restless leg syndrome, are also much more common in subjects with chronic pain compared to the general population. Sleep disturbances are prominent in every central pain disorder, such as fibromyalgia, irritable bowel syndrome, and migraine, as well as in inflammatory and structural pain, including rheumatoid arthritis and osteoarthritis.

Cognitive disturbances are common in chronic pain. This most often involves deficits in attention, executive functioning, and verbal memory. These cognitive disturbances are also strongly correlated with mood and sleep disturbances. Patients with fibromyalgia have described this as "fibro-fog." These cognitive deficits have been well documented with neuropsychological testing, and they are different from those found in dementia. Most importantly, in contrast to dementia, cognitive deficits in chronic pain can be reversed with optimal pain management.

Our thoughts strongly affect our levels of pain. Anticipation and expectations modify how we respond to a painful stimulus. Feeling anxious and worried, particularly when we catastrophize, greatly increases our pain levels. Chronic pain is stressful, and stress releases the "fight or flight" hormones, such as cortisol and epinephrine. When persistently activated, these hormones cause more pain, exhaustion, and insomnia. The impact of prior experiences with pain can be long-lasting.

Neuroimaging has also broadened our understanding of the influence of emotions and mood on chronic pain. We can now visualize the intricate inner connections of brain regions and networks that intermingle pain, sleep, and cognition. When people catastrophize their pain, they feel helpless, and their pain response increases. There are subsequent functional and structural changes in brain areas that influence pain anticipation and perception. For example, the likelihood of phantom limb pain developing following an amputation correlates with an individual's preexisting pain and mood, as well as with catastrophizing.[10] In contrast, when chronic pain is linked to positive emotions and a sense of control, pain levels fall.

Our individual pain sensitivity has genetic influences and therefore is, to some degree, preset. Yet pain responses can vary dramatically, especially with our attention or conditioning. There are plenty of examples of people's transient blotting out of pain. Consider the football player who runs fifty yards for a touchdown with a broken foot and then collapses in agony once the endorphin high ends. Physical and mental conditioning can greatly temper even long-term pain response. Think about the yogi walking across hot coals or the ballerina on pointe, not noticing her tortured, cramped toes.

The cognitive and emotional components of pain are malleable and can be manipulated and modified. Pain relief from distraction or placebo work in identical fashion. The placebo effect is a good example of how thoughts can influence pain response. A placebo is any agent or intervention that is considered to be medically inactive. Placebos are used in clinical trials to determine the efficacy of any treatment. For example, to get a new drug approved for the treatment of any chronic pain disorder, subjects are randomly assigned to receive the active drug or an identical-looking placebo (sugar pill). The subject and examiner are "blinded" as to what each person is receiving. To be approved, the study drug must be significantly more beneficial than the placebo.

However, it has long been known that our individual expectations of pain relief greatly modify our pain reactions. In 1801 John Haygarth wrote that "the passions of the mind had a wonderful and powerful influence upon the state and disorder of the body."[11] Indeed, the placebo effect is harnessed in every successful medical encounter. Having trust and confidence in your health-care provider goes a long way. Experimentally, it was found that if patients received a pain medication from their physician, they experienced significantly more pain relief than when the same medication was provided via a computer-based system, lacking any human contact.[12]

Patient anticipation, modified by verbal or visual cues, greatly influences one's pain reactivity to placebo. In one study looking at the potential benefits of a placebo, half the subjects first were told by doctors that the placebo was likely beneficial while the other subjects received no such suggestion.[13] The subjects who received the pretreatment positive statements reported 50 percent improvement in pain after they took the placebo, compared to only 9 percent improvement in the other group given the identical placebo.

Brain mechanisms activated during the placebo response mirror those of central sensitization. In 1978 it was shown that the placebo effect involves the brain's internal opioid system.[14] Resting-state brain connectivity improves following placebo therapy, correlating with less pain.

Looking at chronic pain through a mind-and-body perspective allows us to better appreciate the complicated relationship between injury, or damage, and pain. In conditions such as fibromyalgia, there is little evidence for muscle or nerve damage and no indication of tissue injury. Treatment directed at damaged muscles or nerves would likely be of little help. In contrast, a person with advanced knee osteoarthritis is likely to have marked pain relief following a knee replacement. Yet the efficacy of that joint replacement may vary substantially based on individual genetic and psychosocial factors. Another example of the complicated interplay of mind and body on chronic pain involves physical trauma, such as a motor vehicle accident (MVA). Persistent pain following an MVA correlates better with social-cultural factors, including preexisting pain, mood, and socioeconomic disadvantage, than with the severity of the crash.[15]

Janet had all the manifestations of fibromyalgia. She was relieved to learn that she wasn't imagining or overreacting and that her pain was real. Her neck and arm pain were aggravated by a pinched nerve and responded well to massage, physical therapy, and exercise. Medications to treat her fibromyalgia also helped her sleep and alleviated her cognitive disturbances. Janet still has flare-ups of her pain, particularly when she is under stress. When these happen, she quickly reevaluates her level of anxiety and discusses this with her therapist.

IMPORTANT POINTS ABOUT MIND AND BODY

- Chronic pain never stems from just mind or just body but always involves both.
- Central nervous system neuroplasticity underlies chronic pain.
- The biopsychological illness model explains the near-universal association of depression with pain.
- Sleep and cognitive disturbances correlate with pain severity and concurrent mood disturbances.

3

NATURE OR NURTURE, AND THE GENDER GAP

Just about every chronic illness is equally influenced by our heredity and our environment. Chronic pain is no exception: 50 percent nature and 50 percent nurture. Looking first at heredity, there are a few, rare chronic pain conditions caused by a single genetic mutation. The best-studied one is the congenital, complete absence of pain. Children with this inherited condition are plagued by constant injury, trauma, and infections that often lead to early death. A British geneticist, Dr. Geoffrey Woods, was the first to identify a mutation in the SCN9A gene that causes congenital pain insensitivity.[1]

Pain-sensing electrical signals to the brain are generated by calcium channels produced by this gene. The SCN9A mutation prevents the gene from making these channels, resulting in loss of normal pain-warning messaging. On November 15, 2012, the *New York Times* featured an article entitled "The Hazards of Growing Up Painlessly," discussing a thirteen-year-old in Georgia, Ashlyn Blocker, born with congenital pain insensitivity.[2] Ashlyn and her family consulted with a colleague of mine, Dr. Roland Staud, a rheumatologist doing pain research at the University of Florida, and Roland found mutations in her SCN9A gene. Roland said, "Her story offers an amazing snapshot of how complicated a life can get without the guidance of pain." Ashlyn's tale of pain insensitivity became a media sensation, and she and her parents appeared on *Today*, *Good Morning America*, and *Inside Edition*; on French TV; and on the BBC. She described putting her hands in boiling water at age two—the flesh burned off without her feeling a twinge of pain—and the time she broke her ankle and ran around on it for a few days without any discomfort.

Other genetic mutations causing pain insensitivity are more subtle. A London geneticist, Dr. James Cox, recently found that a mutation in a gene called FAAH-OUT causes moderate pain insensitivity and is also associated with a flattening of one's mood, to the point of indifference.[3] This genetic flaw exemplifies the universal link of pain with mood.

Apart from these rare genetic defects, the hereditary influences on chronic pain susceptibility are more complex and not related to any single DNA mutation. Family studies, especially those involving twins, have demonstrated genetic risk factors for every chronic pain disorder. Twin studies typically compare monozygotic twins, who share 100 percent of their genes, to dizygotic twins, who share 50 percent of their genes. Comparing the prevalence of a chronic pain condition, like fibromyalgia or migraine, in monozygotic and dizygotic twins allows investigators to unscramble the genetic and environmental factors that impact on that disorder.

Advances in genetic testing, which skyrocketed with the mapping of the human genome, have identified a large number of genes that contribute to pain sensitivity. We now know that the human genome has many genetic variants, the majority called "germline mutations," passed on from parent to children. Some genetic mutations are not inherited and show up only in offspring. These include the SCN9A mutation that causes congenital insensitivity to pain. However, most of the genetic variability in chronic pain conditions does not involve high-impact genes, such as SCN9A, but rather relates to mutations in single nucleotide polymorphisms (SNPs), which are present in more than 1 percent of the general population. Such mutations have a minor impact on disease susceptibility, and their influence is modified by environmental factors—thus nature and nurture acting in concert.

In chronic pain disorders, one of the best studied of these SNPs is the gene that controls the enzyme catechol-O-methyltransferase (COMT), which breaks down neurotransmitters, including epinephrine, norepinephrine, and dopamine. COMT was initially found to strongly influence experimental pain sensitivity and then noted to impact susceptibility for chronic pain disorders, including temporomandibular joint disorder and fibromyalgia.[4] The COMT gene also has a profound influence on the odds of an individual developing chronic pain following a motor vehicle accident. Serotonin transporter genes, first identified as important in depression susceptibility, are also involved in chronic pain predisposition. Opioid-receptor genes and genes that affect inflammation have been linked to a genetic susceptibility to pain. Migraine has been associated with genes involved in neurotransmission, including glutamine, serotonin, and dopamine signaling, pathways critical to pain processing.[5]

In each of the common chronic pain disorders, the genetic influence on pain is intricately tied up with environmental factors. The study of this interplay is termed "epigenetics," wherein heritable changes occur in gene expression without alterations in the underlying DNA sequence.[6] In other words, our basic genetic inheritance pattern is unchanged, but how human traits express themselves is altered by such lifestyle factors as stress and diet. In particular, the strong association of depression and anxiety with chronic pain alters gene expression, termed "DNA methylation."[7] This, in turn, activates stress hormones, leading to a cycle of heightened pain and stress reactivity. Epigenetics fits the biopsychological illness model, explaining how a seemingly fixed trait, like our genetic makeup, is modified by our environment.

At a societal level, socioeconomic factors drive chronic pain. Epidemiological studies of every chronic pain condition have found a strong correlation of low income, less education, and poor working conditions with increased pain severity. For example, African Americans and Hispanics suffer more severe and debilitating pain than whites do.[8] Racial discrimination, with its economic and educational inequities, results in chronic stress, anxiety, frustration, and depression. Individuals living in poor areas are twice as likely to develop chronic pain as those in more affluent areas.

In any one individual, the environmental factors that produce the most profound effect on pain involve stress and mood vulnerability, often called "affective distress." And these begin in childhood. Our physical, emotional, and cognitive reactions to pain are learned early in life and determine how we cope with chronic pain as adults. Parental anxiety and temperament and the way parents themselves react to pain set the pattern for a child's future pain reactivity. Physical and/or sexual abuse as well as a serious illness or hospitalization during childhood are strongly associated with a propensity to chronic pain.

Risk factors for children to develop fibromyalgia as adults include physical, verbal, or sexual abuse; parental depression; divorce; financial problems; serious family illness; and alcohol problems in the family.[9] The association of stress and pain needs to be understood from both a societal and a biological basis. Many patients with fibromyalgia, irritable bowel syndrome, and migraine have a history of post-traumatic stress disorder (PTSD).[10] For example, in one study, 3 percent of the general population had PTSD, but 50 percent of fibromyalgia patients had PTSD.[11] One of the ways in which chronic stress leads to chronic pain involves the hypothalamic-pituitary-adrenal (HPA) axis, our stress hormonal system. Investigators in the UK followed subjects from the general population over a number of years, confirming the importance of psychosocial risk factors on developing chronic, widespread pain.[12] At baseline, they measured the subjects' stress response by experimental stimulation of the HPA axis. They found that the odds of developing chronic, widespread pain later in life correlated with the severity of the HPA-axis reactivity.

Many of the environmental risk factors for chronic pain, such as socioeconomic status, are difficult to alter. Others, such as diet and lifestyle, can be individually modified. Multiple studies have found that obesity, smoking, lack of exercise, and inactivity are risk factors for chronic pain. All of these environmental influences are interrelated.

Often the nature-or-nurture argument is misunderstood. If we think that our chronic pain is predetermined, we may feel helpless to alter its course. Following a recent medical review article on fibromyalgia that I wrote, a distraught reader sent me a letter, troubled by my statement that obesity is a risk factor for chronic pain and that treatment should include weight reduction and exercise. She admonished me for not explaining that both fibromyalgia and obesity are determined by genetic factors and have identical hereditary abnormalities. I was less troubled by the fact that she erroneously believed there to be a known genetic link between obesity and fibromyalgia than by how she was misinterpreting that possibility. Even if such a link were found, this does not mean that attempts at weight reduction and exercise would be doomed to failure. Each of us can modify lifestyle factors that promote chronic pain.

As discussed in the previous chapter, emotions greatly influence pain. Depression, anxiety, and fear activate stress, which in turn triggers pain. If these persist, neural remapping fosters pain hypersensitivity. My patients have often described an exacerbation of their pain following a stressful event. Recognizing this flare-up as a normal physiologic response reassures them that it is likely to be transient. If we feel helpless and hopeless, we are unable to focus on anything but our pain. Our thoughts are consumed with, Why me? Will I ever get better? We can lose our self-worth, our identity. Often we become angry and seek retribution.

The gender gap in chronic pain also involves inherited (sex-related, i.e., chromosomal) and environmental factors. Women have a lower pain tolerance than men do for a variety of noxious stimuli.[13] Every chronic pain condition is more common in women than in men. In most fibromyalgia studies, the ratio of females to males is about four to one. In migraine the ratio is three to one, in complex regional pain it is also three to one, and in irritable bowel syndrome it is two to one. What accounts for this female predominance?

Dr. William Maixner, a pain researcher at the University of North Carolina, surmised that females have evolved heightened sensations, not only for pain but also for smell, temperature, and visual cues.[14] This evolution is gender-specific. Sex hormones, such as testosterone and progesterone, influence stress and pain reactivity in humans and other mammals. This was initially noted in fruit flies and birds. Subsequently these sex differences were noted in most species. Female rodents have a lower experimental pain threshold to pressure, heat, and chemical stimuli. As in human studies, this correlates with a more robust stress response in female rodents. Such sex hormone influences help explain why some women have attacks of migraine only during their menstrual cycle and why migraine often disappears with the onset of menopause. Genetic variability interacts with sex hormone status to influence pain sensitivity. A genetic variant of an opioid receptor gene was found to be associated with pain sensitivity in men but not in women.[15] Neuroimaging studies have demonstrated significant gender differences in brain pain-processing regions.

Centuries-old societal roles for masculinity and femininity helped shape the role of gender in chronic pain. Women more often seek social support and are less likely to repress their emotions. Men are told to "toughen up." Women are more likely to visit a physician and more likely to report pain as a symptom than men are. Men more often use problem-focused techniques and behavior distraction when dealing with chronic pain. Women tend to be more self-analytic.

Such gender role bias has fostered unfortunate stereotypes regarding women with chronic pain. Throughout the 1800s the fashionable term for fibromyalgia and chronic fatigue was "neurasthenia," or nervous exhaustion.[16] This was thought to be related to a "depletion of our limited supply of nervous energy," more common in women in Western society who were facing heightened stress in an industrialized world. When neurasthenia became prominent in large segments of society, it was often attributed to a form of mass hysteria, almost exclusively in women. "Hysteria" comes from the Greek word for uterus and has been applied almost always to women.

Author Virginia Woolf, sexually abused during her youth, suffered from recurrent bouts of depression and was diagnosed by her Harley Street, London, physicians with neurasthenia. Woolf described her prolonged episodes of exhaustion, headaches, and insomnia in her essay "On Being Ill."[17] Woolf was told to avoid any physical or mental exertion and to retire to bed in a dark room. She was often considered to be hysterical. Woolf's father also suffered from chronic headaches, insomnia, depression, and anxiety, suggesting a genetic link to neurasthenia. Today we would classify patients with neurasthenia as having fibromyalgia or chronic fatigue syndrome.

In contrast, men returning from war exhibiting symptoms that now would be diagnosed as fibromyalgia and chronic fatigue were said to be suffering from shell shock, battle fatigue, or, later on, Gulf War syndrome. About one-third of veterans of the Gulf War complain of chronic pain, fatigue, headaches, depression, and cognitive disturbances.[18] The diagnostic label Gulf War syndrome implied, without good evidence, that exposure to toxins of war caused the chronic pain and suffering. Medical and societal empathy for these male-dominant syndromes are much greater than those for similar female-dominant syndromes, such as neurasthenia, fibromyalgia, or chronic fatigue syndrome.

Gender selection bias and stereotypes have adversely affected medical research in chronic pain. In both animal and human studies, the vast majority of subjects have been males. Dr. Daniela Pollak, a neurobiologist, wrote in a review article on sex and gender bias, "We live in a world where the assumption is that males are the standard, the reference population, and females are the ones that are odd."[19] We now know that women get less pain relief from opioid and anti-inflammatory medications than men do, yet gender is never taken into account when doctors prescribe medications for chronic pain. Research in pain needs to recognize the importance of gender.

These unfortunate gender stereotypes persist. When I was recently discussing the reasons why fibromyalgia is diagnosed more often in women, a rheumatologist snickered that "after all, it is a female condition." I knew he was implying "the weaker sex." Gender differences in chronic pain, like genetic and epigenetic factors, are equally the product of nature and nurture. Implying that it's all nature is fatalistic. Suggesting that it's all related to our environment fosters harmful labeling and stereotypes, such as passing off chronic pain in women as exaggerated or hysterical. Chronic pain is determined jointly by what lies inside and outside of our being.

IMPORTANT POINTS ABOUT NATURE AND NURTURE

- Chronic pain is determined equally by hereditary and environmental forces.
- Risk factors, particularly stress, are predictors of chronic pain and can be modified.
- Women are more susceptible to chronic pain; this is determined in part by intrinsic factors and fostered by attitudes and beliefs.
- Gender is important in pain sensitivity and diagnostic labeling and must be taken into account in research and in treatment regarding all forms of chronic pain.

4

PAIN EDUCATION AND MISINFORMATION

Scott's first severe headache occurred just after he had finished running in a high school cross-country meet. His description of that headache matched my own experience, including the visual aura and the throbbing over his forehead and temple. Over the next ten years he went to many headache specialists and tried various medications but continued to suffer from frequent headaches. In college he spent a lot of time searching the internet for headache remedies and joined online headache support groups.

Much of the internet-derived information focused on the role of various foods and diet in migraine. Scott tried low-sodium, sugar-free, and gluten-free diets. Websites and patient blogs extolled the benefits of nutraceuticals, such as feverfew and butterbur extract, both used by Scott with no benefit. Over the past few years, Scott joined five different migraine social networks. The attacks of migraine persisted.

Despite the fact that chronic pain is the most common health condition in the United States, there is an alarming lack of public pain education. Only 18 percent of Americans identified chronic pain as a major public health problem, compared to 50 percent identifying drug addiction, 37 percent alcoholism, and 34 percent Alzheimer's disease.[1] Yet each of these conditions is much less common and less costly than chronic pain. A national task force noted that most Americans have little understanding of the distinction between acute and chronic pain or that pain can be a disease in its own right.[2]

Today most people utilize the internet when seeking health information. There are more than seventy thousand websites offering health advice.[3] More than two-thirds of internet users seek medical information online, usually at least once each month.[4] This has provided the public with a wealth of medical information at their fingertips at no significant cost and in the privacy of their own home. In our current medical system, health-care providers can't keep up with the pace of new medical information, there is less time to spend with patients for discussing potential new data, and there is a burgeoning public interest in alternative health care.

The internet has provided the public with widespread access to health information. However, the quality of that health information is often poor.[5] Internet medical advice varies from extremely useful to downright dangerous, all depending on who provides the information.[6] A spokesperson for the US Department of Health and Human Services said, "Trying to get information from the Internet is like drinking from a firehose, and you don't even know what the source of the water is."[7] Despite this, 50 percent of consumers report that online health-care information influenced their treatment decisions.[8] As internet health information expands exponentially, there is a danger of information overload, and it becomes ever more difficult to find what is most relevant.

Internet websites that promote their own products have been consistently rated as providing the most inaccurate and incomplete health-care information. Websites sponsored by universities, medical schools, and recognized research centers and hospitals, and government-sponsored sites, like those provided by the National Institutes of Health (NIH), offer the best quality.[9] Most professional organizations offer reliable information although bias is more likely.

There is no gold standard for evaluating health information on the Web. One study utilized an expert panel to compare website information on fibromyalgia.[10] Of the most popular twenty-five websites, ten were nonprofit but six were commercial. The average score for accuracy and completeness was 2.5 out of 5. The top-rated websites were sponsored by the NIH or other medical institutions. Another survey found that less than 50 percent of sixty websites on low back pain provided reliable medical information.[11] Websites with commercial sponsorship provided the poorest quality health information.

The websites that I routinely recommend to my fibromyalgia patients are sponsored by the Arthritis Foundation, the Centers for Disease Control (CDC), and the American College of Rheumatology. The FibroGuide site, sponsored by the University of Michigan Medical Center, provides a comprehensive tutorial on understanding and treating fibromyalgia. These academic-affiliated websites are easy to access and permanent fixtures of the internet, in contrast to many commercial sites, which often disappear.

One in four internet health information seekers will join a support group, either online or in person.[12] Support groups can provide valuable resources for patients, particularly in establishing social support and a sense of community. However, support groups often deliver unbalanced medical guidance when their leaders have a personal agenda and there are no health-care professionals on board. Some of the fibromyalgia support groups that I have encountered dedicated their discussions to getting members disability coverage rather than to ways to manage their condition. Online support groups often promote unconventional remedies.

I was one of the expert physicians who helped Pfizer, the largest pharmaceutical company in the world, design fibromyalgia information websites in conjunction with the launch of their medication, Lyrica (pregabalin). As physician advisors we were careful to avoid promoting the new drug and tried our best to make the website unbiased and replete with useful information on fibromyalgia, including the latest research on the mechanisms of chronic pain. Nevertheless, subtle sponsor-related influences are difficult to escape.

The most popular health information subject, whether accessed from the internet or from ebooks, involves special diets,
supplements, or "natural" therapies. The most popular fibromyalgia websites are all commercial, including one offering "amazing
relief" with a single natural supplement that contains "every B, C
and D vitamin plus Rhodiola, Quercetin, L-Theanine, Tumeric
[sic] root and Zingerber [sic] Officinale, all in one capsule." It
proclaims, "Tons of users reporting stunning results." The five
most popular sites for migraine are either pharmaceutical or com-
mercially sponsored.

Many of the most popular books available online are written by
patients, many of whom have quasi-medical backgrounds. They
typically extol the virtues of their personal pathway to conquering
an illness. A lot of these books are linked to selling a product. This
is the case when looking through the most popular ebooks about
fibromyalgia as well as those related to migraine.

There is no quality filter when accessing the internet or when
joining a support group or when buying a health-related book.
Anyone can develop an internet site, start a support group, or
become an author and publisher. Watch out for medical websites
that don't include author credentials or references to their data
sources. Is the e-book author a health care professional, is there a
product being touted, and do the claims seem outrageous? Is the
work being published by a legitimate publisher, or is it self-pub-
lished through an online platform? Does the work refer to other
studies on the subject, and were these published in peer-reviewed
journals? Is the information based solely on the author's "expertise," garnered though personal experience? Check out the author's online presence and background and, if these are not provided, try to look them up. Be especially skeptical when traditional
medicine is eschewed or outrageous claims or magic cures are
proclaimed. Warning signs include phrases like "scientific break-
through," "exclusive product or recipe," or "secret ingredient."

Another source of medical information and misinformation for
the public is direct-to-consumer advertising (DTCA). During the
first twenty years of my medical career, there was no advertising

by physicians or hospitals, and it was felt that such advertising would undermine our integrity and damage the public trust. In 1997 the FDA approved television and radio marketing by pharma as long as the advertisement struck a balance between a drug's use, its benefits, and its potential harm.[13] Annually more than $10 million is spent on these ads, and the total spending on DTCA has increased 400 percent in the past twenty years.[14]

Pharma claims that these ads raise consumer awareness of health issues. However, there is little educational value provided by DTCA, and its main purpose is to sell a product. DTCA offers little information about disease mechanisms, risk factors, or prevalence. DTCA typically uses broad emotional appeal factors, such as regaining control of your life. Since potential drug harms must be mentioned, a significant amount of airtime is allocated to every conceivable side effect, but the consumer has no way to put this in perspective. Generic medications are never advertised. Pharmaceutical companies plow their money into the promotion of their newest and most expensive products. Pharma drug marketing often makes good use of a viewer's motivation to self-diagnose. Advertisement promotion understands the power of personalizing an illness.[15] A product is likely to be sold when you see yourself in an advertisement. DTCA has resulted in health-care providers prescribing more drugs, and more expensive ones, despite the fact that most physicians believe that DTCA is harmful to the public. The American Medical Association has suggested that DTCA be banned.

Shortly after Lyrica was approved by the FDA for the treatment of fibromyalgia, there were twenty-one different Lyrica advertising spots on various networks. Between 2013 and 2018 these ads aired more than two thousand times nationally. Tabetha Violet, a graduate student researcher, wrote that these advertisements often capitalize on a gender-specific fear of disability.[16] In one ad, a woman with fibromyalgia talks about her pain, her brow furrowed while she rubs her neck and shoulder. Then the screen flips to a body mannequin with "overactive nerves" pulsing in red. Violet notes, "The woman has become disembodied: instead of maintaining her identity, she is now literally transformed into the depiction of her pain."[17] Another commercial depicts a woman standing alone on a dock as her family gets in a canoe and slowly drifts away, the imagery capturing the fear of being left behind. In each advertisement the women are depicted as doing their activities poorly before the medication but doing them well once they start taking the drug. The women are transformed, not only free of pain but also free of social isolation. Every pharmaceutical company pitches its product, but this often results in unrealistic patient expectations. In chronic pain, there are no magic bullets.

The best approach to providing accurate health-care information to the public is for consistent collaboration with their health-care professionals. However, physicians suffer from inadequate pain education and are inundated with misinformation, just as the public is.

Only 4 percent of American medical schools require a course on chronic pain, and only 16 percent have a pain-based elective as part of the curriculum.[18] In physician residency training there is seldom any formal chronic pain education. Eighty percent of primary care providers consider chronic pain to be one of the most challenging conditions to treat but state that it had been a low priority in their medical training.[19] Fewer than 50 percent of US primary care physicians felt at least "somewhat prepared" to handle chronic pain patients.[20] Chronic pain is identified as the condition most likely to make physicians feel helpless in caring for their patients.[21]

Physicians are hardly immune to the health misinformation engendered by pharmaceutical company marketing. DTCA makes up only 15 percent of the $30 billion that pharma spends yearly.[22] The vast majority of that marketing budget is spent on influencing physicians. Much of this money goes to drug company representatives making sales calls to physicians. This is touted by pharma to inform the doctors about a specific drug but has included giving out free samples of the medication as well as meals and gifts. Early in my career, this form of marketing was ubiquitous. Most physicians felt that the benefit from receiving free drugs to give our patients offset any potential bias we might incur. The information about the medication often included a talk by a medical expert along with a sumptuous meal at a fancy restaurant or a conference at a ski or golf resort with the tab picked up by the pharmaceutical representatives. Of course, the medical expert was given a substantial honorarium by the drug company.

Subsequently it was shown that such drug detailing had pervasive effects on physician behavior, with obvious conflicts of interest. Gifts and free meals have largely been prohibited at most hospitals, and educational activities at most medical centers are no longer sponsored by pharma. Curtailing of widespread pharma influence has reduced the likelihood that a physician will prescribe an expensive new medication that has no advantage over existing drugs. However, most practicing physicians still see a pharmaceutical representative regularly and receive free medications, and many still attend industry-sponsored continuing medical education. The result is a subtle conflict of interest. More blatant examples of a health-care provider linked to a commercial product include TV ads that help patients find a doctor or a clinic that offers their product or device. Sometimes you don't even need to see the doctor face-to-face.

As a patient, you will find that pain education will be most accurate and focused when it is from your health-care team and when you openly discuss what you have found on your own. Physicians have access to multiple, high-level sources of patient information, be they pamphlets to hand out or websites to recommend. Patients need to be aware of industry-based payments and potential conflicts of interest.

We need much greater focus on patient and physician pain education, as outlined in the Institute of Medicine's 2011 report: "From initial education through continuing education programs, health professionals need to learn more about the importance of pain prevention, ways to prevent the transition from acute to chronic pain, how to treat pain more effectively and cost-effectively, and how to prevent other physical and psychological conditions associated with pain."[23]

IMPORTANT POINTS ABOUT PAIN EDUCATION AND MISINFORMATION

- There is a lack of public awareness regarding all aspects of chronic pain.
- Most internet medical sites are commercial and lack credible information.
- Health information relying on personal anecdotes, making unusual claims, or touting alternative therapies at the expense of traditional medicine should be avoided.
- Direct-to-consumer advertising uses broad emotional appeal factors, such as regaining control of your life, and typically has little educational value.
- Health-care information is most helpful and accurate when accessed via patient/physician collaboration.
- There is a major gap in current health-care professionals' pain education.

5

FIBROMYALGIA

Patty's fibromyalgia was triggered by the disrupted and fragmented sleep she experienced while recuperating from her traumatic eye injury. Fortuitously, as I began my own research in fibromyalgia, I met Drs. Harvey Moldofsky and Hugh Smythe, who had described sleep disturbances as being very common in patients with fibromyalgia. Smythe, a rheumatologist, and Moldofsky, a psychiatrist, established a sleep laboratory in Toronto and in 1975 published the first human study linking sleep with pain.[1] Medical students slept in their laboratory while hooked up to an electroencephalogram (EEG), which monitored their brain wave activity throughout the night. Human brain wave patterns change during various stages of sleep. Deep, nondream sleep is termed stage 4 and is our most restorative phase of sleep. Whenever the EEG showed the student entering into stage 4 sleep, a buzzer sounded in the laboratory. The noise did not fully awaken the student but was sufficient to cause blips of electrical interference in the EEG, termed alpha wave intrusion into stage 4 sleep. After a few nights of this, the students each complained of fatigue and generalized body pain and were tender to palpation in specific soft-tissue spots. This got many of us thinking that fibromyalgia was caused by disrupted deep sleep.

Unfortunately, it was not that simple. Yes, Patty's pain eased up after her sleep improved with the tiny amount of amitriptyline she began taking nightly. However, her symptoms did not disappear. Furthermore, the alpha wave intrusion in stage 4 sleep was prominent in patients with fibromyalgia but was also noted in many other chronic pain conditions.

Sleep has a profound influence on pain sensitivity and tolerance. Sleep deprivation, as in the medical students, experimentally decreases pain thresholds to pressure, heat, and cold.[2] In a prospective study of twelve thousand women, self-reported sleep disturbances were the most important predictor of developing chronic, widespread pain, but other factors, such as depression, were co-contributors.[3] Poor sleep, like depression, predisposes to chronic pain, and they typically occur together.[4] However, chronic pain is not simply a sleep disorder.

We still could not pinpoint the root cause of fibromyalgia. Back in the early 1800s fibromyalgia had been called "fibrositis" and was thought to be caused by subtle inflammation in peripheral nerves and soft tissues, as described in 1841 by Valleix: "If it remains concentrated in the nerves, one finds characteristic, isolated, painful points. This is neuralgia in the proper sense. If the pain spreads into the muscles, the muscular contractions are principally painful. This is muscular rheumatism."[5] During the next century, investigators were unable to find evidence for any nerve or tissue inflammation or injury. Physicians haven't given up on the notion that damaged nerves trigger fibromyalgia, and some believe that fibromyalgia is often caused by a small fiber neuropathy. However, a peripheral neuropathy would not explain the widespread body pain, exhaustion, and sleep and mood disturbances characteristic of fibromyalgia.

Since the early 1980s most fibromyalgia researchers have been seeking answers in the brain. Fibromyalgia skeptics pounced upon this, thinking that the fibromyalgia "experts" had finally come around to the idea that "it is all in the head." This fit with many medical journals and textbooks lumping fibromyalgia into mental disorders dubbed "psychogenic rheumatism." Fibromyalgia, chronic headaches, and irritable bowel syndrome were each called "psychosomatic," a term invented by psychiatrists. It implied that psychological states, such as anxiety and depression, were being expressed by physical symptoms, including chronic pain—again, the mind or body, rather than the mind *and* the body.

Genetic and environmental factors work in concert to raise the odds of anyone getting fibromyalgia. Fibromyalgia is eight times more likely to develop if a parent has the condition.[6] Although no single gene can explain this familial predisposition, there are a number of genetic factors that contribute to fibromyalgia susceptibility. Fibromyalgia may be triggered by physical or emotional trauma and is much more common when this trauma occurs in childhood, such as with physical or sexual abuse.[7]

Neck injury, such as the result of a motor vehicle accident (MVA), and repeated physical and emotional trauma in the workplace have been associated with fibromyalgia. However, it has been difficult to separate out these physical events from associated psychosocial factors. For example, the presence of persistent pain after an MVA was more strongly associated with preexisting depression and patient catastrophizing than with collision factors, such as vehicle damage or type of collision.[8] Individuals engaged in post-MVA litigation had significantly greater odds of developing fibromyalgia than nonlitigants. In the workplace, certain mechanical factors, such as prolonged work with one's hands at or above shoulder level, increase the risk of fibromyalgia. Low job satisfaction and monotonous work were even greater predictors of fibromyalgia developing in the workplace. Nearly 50 percent of female veterans have fibromyalgia symptoms. The presence and severity of these symptoms correlated with a past medical history of depression, post-traumatic stress disorder (PTSD), and sexual trauma.

Alcoholism, cigarette smoking, lack of exercise, and obesity are risk factors for fibromyalgia. Here, too, it is difficult to separate these issues from one another and from shared social influences, such as education and income. Individual personality traits also predict the likelihood of fibromyalgia. Catastrophizing correlates with the prevalence and severity of fibromyalgia.[9] In contrast, self-efficacy has been an important predictor of a better fibromyalgia outcome.

These external and internal driving forces set in motion the central sensitization that perpetuates chronic pain. Early fibromyalgia studies demonstrated aberrant levels of pain substances, such as substance P (P for pain) in the cerebrospinal fluid.[10] More recently, neuroimaging has provided investigators with a tool to study pain mechanisms in experimental models and to follow changes over time in patients with fibromyalgia. Following a modest amount of pressure applied to the forearm, fibromyalgia patients had significantly greater pain than did healthy subjects.[11] MRIs on the fibromyalgia patients revealed much greater activity in brain regions that transmit pain sensations. Fibromyalgia patients also exhibited more catastrophizing behavior than control subjects, and this correlated with greater neuronal activity in pain regions of their brains.

Neuroimaging studies have demonstrated brain structural alterations, such as loss of gray matter, in fibromyalgia.[12] These structural changes correlated with the duration and severity of pain. Elevated levels of neurotransmitters, such as glutamate, are present in the insula of fibromyalgia patients compared to healthy controls. Even at rest, changes have been found in the brains of fibromyalgia patients, such as altered connectivity between pain-connecting regions. Fibromyalgia is now considered to be the prototypical centralized pain disorder with pain originating in the central nervous system.

Rather than searching for a single cause of fibromyalgia, we now focus on triggering, aggravating, and perpetuating factors. Some of these are fixed, while others can be modified. Some are internal, while others are external. Sorting this all out is not easy, neither for fibromyalgia patients nor their health-care providers.

What have the past forty years taught us about a diagnosis of fibromyalgia? My early rheumatology training reflected the widely held belief that the pain and other physical complaints of fibromyalgia did not fit any disease pattern. It was a "wastebasket" diagnosis, not a distinct medical condition. Once I became involved in fibromyalgia research, I had a heated public debate with a prominent rheumatologist who said, "Fibromyalgia is not real, in contrast to rheumatoid arthritis."[13] That opinion changed after a number of my colleagues and I published an article in our premier rheumatology journal suggesting that fibromyalgia was a discrete illness that could be diagnosed easily by a careful history and a physical examination.[14]

The diagnosis of fibromyalgia is based on widespread, chronic pain throughout the body that can't be attributed to any other medical disorder.[15] As described by Patty, patients commonly state, "It feels like I always have the flu." Fibromyalgia is almost always associated with exhaustion and sleep disturbances. Most often the sleep is light and unrefreshing. Fibromyalgia patients often comment, like Patty, "I can barely get out of bed and feel so exhausted, like I was run over by a truck." Sometimes fibromyalgia patients will have a primary sleep disturbance such as sleep apnea or restless leg syndrome. If a patient reports persistent, widespread body pain for at least three months, along with fatigue and sleep disturbances, and the physician excludes other medical causes of the chronic pain, the fibromyalgia diagnosis is very likely.

A confusing aspect of fibromyalgia relates to its multitude of symptoms including bowel, bladder, and pelvic pain, chronic headaches, and jaw and facial pain, all of which afflicted Patty. Somewhere between 30 and 60 percent of fibromyalgia patients will be diagnosed with irritable bowel syndrome, chronic pelvic/bladder pain, or temporomandibular joint syndrome, as will be subsequently discussed.[16]

Fibromyalgia diagnostic criteria have allowed investigators to make a number of important conclusions regarding this chronic pain condition. Fibromyalgia is very common, affecting 3 to 8 percent of the population. The prevalence varies based on what criteria have been used in epidemiologic surveys. In some studies, fibromyalgia and chronic, widespread pain (CWP) are considered the same condition. In most countries throughout the world, CWP affects 10 to 15 percent of the population. Fibromyalgia and CWP are twice as common in females and present in all age groups throughout the world, with no major ethnic propensity. Fibromyalgia is also common in patients with rheumatic diseases, occurring in 20 to 40 percent of patients with osteoarthritis, rheumatoid arthritis, systemic lupus erythematosus, Sjogren's syndrome, and ankylosing spondylitis. Rheumatologists now recognize the importance of determining whether an exacerbation of pain in these diseases is related to active joint inflammation or concomitant fibromyalgia.

Despite the general recognition of fibromyalgia as an important medical condition, it continues to generate diagnostic controversy and confusion. Echoing earlier sentiments that it is not real or not a discrete illness, some believe that the fibromyalgia diagnosis feeds into illness behavior. They claim that every human being suffers from body pain, soreness, exhaustion, and insomnia at times and that giving these symptoms a diagnostic label "medicalizes" the complaints. Once assigned a medical diagnosis, one seeks more medical attention, sees more medical specialists, and sees oneself as a patient rather than a person with everyday symptoms.

Such a downward spiral can happen if the diagnosis of fibromyalgia is not accompanied by a comprehensive discussion about what the condition is or isn't. If the patient is not reassured, there will be worry about a missed diagnosis, like systemic lupus erythematosus or Lyme disease. Costly and invasive tests and multiple specialist referrals ensue, leading to heightened diagnostic uncertainty and anxiety. The average time to make a diagnosis of fibromyalgia is greater than three years.[17]

Fibromyalgia is associated with depression and anxiety. Often it is hard to know what came first. Fibromyalgia patients worry that their doctor will presume that it is all in their head. It is important that health-care providers, patients, and their family do not get the message that fibromyalgia is the same thing as depression. All forms of chronic pain are associated with depression, and there are genetic and biologic similarities. Some physicians classify fibromyalgia as a psychosomatic disorder. After all, patients look fine, and their laboratory tests and X-rays are normal. Since there is no organic disease, it must be in the patient's imagination or psyche.

Doctors often make light of fibromyalgia. Even today, medical students and trainees get the message that fibromyalgia is not legitimate or important since it is rarely featured in their training. A review of medical students' attitudes toward fibromyalgia was titled "If It's a Medical Issue I Would Have Covered It by Now."[18] Quotes from the students included these:

"I think there is a general lack of training about it."
"I think doctors do what they can, but they don't seem to know very much about it."
"Perhaps with no teaching on fibromyalgia, then you think that it's not as prominent or not as important to learn about."

As a faculty member at Oregon Health Sciences University, I have had the opportunity to teach a course on fibromyalgia and chronic pain to the medical students and residents. Their concerns and comments about chronic pain and its management reflect those of physicians everywhere. Typical comments include, "Is it a medical or psychiatric disorder? How can I be sure I am not missing something? These patients are so difficult to treat that I dread taking care of them."

Some physicians are not comfortable with the waxing and waning nature of fibromyalgia symptoms. Fibromyalgia can morph diagnostically from a trait or a state to a disease. Some of us are genetically predisposed to the trait of fibromyalgia. Depending on environmental stressors, a transient state of fibromyalgia can emerge. However, once the symptoms reach a certain severity and level of persistence, fibromyalgia or chronic pain becomes a disease. My depression was transient; I am no longer depressed. My migraine comes and goes. Patty is doing so well that she would currently not fulfill the diagnostic criteria for fibromyalgia.

The recognition that fibromyalgia was a recognizable illness with diagnostic criteria allowed clinicians to test various treatment regimens in reliable studies, so-called randomized controlled trials

(RCTs). One of the initial studies was by our group in Boston demonstrating that 25 mg of amitriptyline given at bedtime, the same medication I used to treat Patty, performed significantly better than placebo in fibromyalgia patients. Subsequently, RCTs led to the FDA approval of Lyrica (pregabalin); Cymbalta (duloxetine); and Savella (milnacipran), for the treatment of fibromyalgia in the United States. Controlled studies then demonstrated the efficacy of exercise and various nonpharmacologic therapies in patients with fibromyalgia.

On September 14, 2017, Lady Gaga released a statement to the press canceling her worldwide tour because she was "suffering from severe physical pain that . . . impacted her ability to perform," and shortly thereafter admitted that she had been diagnosed with fibromyalgia.[19] A few months later, Netflix released Lady Gaga's documentary film, *Gaga, Five Foot Two*, which I scrutinized from a professional and personal perspective.

When I first listened to Lady Gaga's musical hits, I thought her to be a rather outrageous performer, better suited to my grandchildren's taste than mine, but over the years I grew to appreciate her enormous talent and charisma. Viewing her documentary, I was interested in learning how one of the most famous celebrities in the world was dealing with fibromyalgia. Even with her wealth and fame, getting a correct diagnosis took Lady Gaga much too long. She noted, "I have chased this pain for the past five years."[20]

Like Patty with her eye injury, Lady Gaga thought that her fibromyalgia began with a hip injury. About 50 percent of patients with fibromyalgia date the onset of their chronic pain to physical or emotional trauma. In the film, she described the impact of mood and stress on her pain: "If I get depressed, my body goes into spasm . . . and I have had body pain, fear, paranoia, and anxiety for the past five years."[21] This is depicted as we observe her during a severe pain flare-up, crying in agony, precipitated by the stress of preparing for her Super Bowl halftime performance in 2017. Despite being enormously successful and adored, Lady Gaga acknowledges her insecurity and lack of self-efficacy, a common trait in people with chronic pain: "I was never pretty enough or good enough . . . I can never get it all right at the same time."[22]

During the film Lady Gaga is seen in treatment with her physician, a specialist in physical medicine and rehabilitation. The doctor discusses the importance of psychological management as well as an array of physical therapies. We observe Lady Gaga receiving deep tissue massage, acupuncture, and injections into soft-tissue areas and watch her doing a series of exercises designed to stretch and loosen her taut muscles. Lady Gaga addresses the lack of public information and health-care interest and funding for chronic pain conditions like fibromyalgia, and she wishes "to help raise awareness and connect people who have it."[23] We need more celebrities like Lady Gaga to acknowledge fibromyalgia as real and to help pursue research for a clearer understanding and better management of this common cause of chronic pain.

Like Patty, Lady Gaga suffered from an invisible illness. Patients with fibromyalgia always look healthy, so how can they be so ill? This is the quandary in most chronic pain conditions. You can't see it, tests don't show it, so how do your doctors, family, and friends believe you? The diagnosis of invisible chronic pain like fibromyalgia can be especially challenging for patients and health-care professionals. We have come a long way in the past twenty years, and fibromyalgia is now generally accepted as a discrete illness with reliable diagnostic criteria. We still have a long way to go to improve its early recognition, to dissuade people that it is "all in the head," and to discover more effective therapy.

FIBROMYALGIA DIAGNOSIS

- Chronic, widespread pain
- Exhaustion, sleep disturbances, mood disturbances
- Normal routine tests; lack of outward signs
- Overlap with other chronic pain conditions like headaches; bowel, pelvic, and bladder pain

FIBROMYALGIA TREATMENT

- Patient and family education
- Treatment for insomnia
- Activity and exercise
- Stress reduction, relaxation, mindfulness
- Trial with a medication such as amitriptyline, duloxetine, or pregabalin

6

MIGRAINE

My first attack of migraine occurred when I was in my late twenties. It began with double vision, but within seconds I saw flashing lines and strange shapes that obscured my sight. This ushered in the worst headache of my life. It began on the right side of my temple and quickly spread to my forehead and down the right side of my face. At the time, I was at work and I had to excuse myself and lie down. I was unable to see patients for the rest of the afternoon. I took a bunch of aspirin and shut my eyes and learned over the years that this was the quickest way to get rid of the headaches.

Ever since then I have been plagued by migraine about once a month. My migraine always begins with visual aura. Aura, derived from the Greek word for "breeze," is a transient neurologic event. Now I don't panic, because I know the aura will go away within thirty minutes, often without any headache, if I immediately take three ibuprofen or three aspirin, lie down, and shut my eyes. Migraine without the headache is termed an ocular migraine. However, if I don't catch the migraine in time, I can be laid up for hours with a headache and seemingly unrelated systemic and psychologic symptoms. That is classic migraine. When there is no aura, it is termed "common migraine."

The visual symptoms are the most striking manifestation of the migraine aura. The visual aura may include flashes of colors, often mixed together, giving the appearance of a rainbow. These can coalesce into a brilliant mosaic. Other visual phenomena include fortification spectra, looking like walls of a fort or castle, zigzag lines, and elaborate figures, which can be quite frightening. Another common visual aura, termed "scintillating scotoma," is a flickering alteration in or total loss of portions of the visual field. Although the auras, like mine, are most often composed of visual phenomena, they can include various symptoms, such as numbness and tingling, intense sounds, altered taste sensations, and even loss of consciousness.

The typical migraine headache is on one side of the head, most severe around the temple and forehead, and throbbing in nature. The headaches are also frequently described as stabbing or aching. Any activity aggravates the headache, as do bright lights, hence the universal advice that I follow: to lie down, eyes shut, in a dark room. Untreated the average migraine lasts up to twelve hours, with almost 50 percent recurring within the next day or two.

Migraine affects 10 to 20 percent of people, a billion worldwide.[1] It is more common in women and usually begins between the ages of twenty and forty. Migraine was accurately characterized by Hippocrates two thousand years ago.[2] The term *migraine* was coined by the Roman physician Galen from the word "hemicrania," since the headaches usually involve one side of the face and head.

Migraine has affected many illustrious historical figures including Julius Caesar, Sigmund Freud, Elvis Presley, and John Kennedy. Rudyard Kipling elegantly described his hemicrania: "One half of my head in a mathematical line from the top of my skull to the cleft of my jaw, throbs and hammers and sizzles and bangs and swears."[3] Lewis Carroll, the author of *Alice in Wonderland*, suffered from severe migraine.[4] Carroll, the pen name of Charles Dodgson, based Alice's hallucinatory travels down the rabbit hole, dubbed "Alice in Wonderland syndrome," on the visual fantasies he experienced during his migraine. Carroll drew figures in his sketchbook of a man standing, with parts of his face, shoulder, and arm missing on the right side, apparently similar to what he visualized during a visual aura scotoma.[5]

Although much less common than tension or muscle headaches, migraine is typically more debilitating and associated with the widest array of physical and psychologic symptoms. It is the sixth most common cause of worldwide disability.[6] There is also an infinite number of variations, presentations, and severity of these symptoms. My migraine is always associated with nausea. Dizziness often accompanies the aura. Many people experience more severe gastrointestinal symptoms with migraine, including abdominal pain, diarrhea, sweating, and facial flushing. Mood disturbances and exhaustion are prominent with migraine headaches. During migraines, or more commonly just after the pain subsides, there is intense lethargy and depression although some patients suffer with severe anxiety and irritability.[7]

There are striking similarities between migraine and fibromyalgia, including historical perspectives, potential causal or triggering factors, role of gender, and the associated physical and psychological symptoms. Ancient Greek and Roman physicians thought migraine to be caused by evil humors, or circulating hormones, arising from the uterus.[8] The Greek word for uterus, *hystera*, then became associated with a migraine personality, often thought of as hysteria. Trepanation, drilling of holes into the skull to allow those evil humors to escape, was a common migraine treatment, even advocated by Dr. William Harvey in the seventeenth century.[9] A stereotype migraine patient was seen as a thin, pale, worried-looking female, often obsessive and perfectionistic. In Victorian times migraine, like fibromyalgia, was lumped under the medical disorder of neurasthenia.[10]

More than three hundred years ago, Thomas Willis described the potential precipitating events that migraine sufferers report: "An evil or weak constitution, sometimes innate and hereditary, an irritation in some distant viscera, changes of season, violent passions and errors in diet, all might bring on the attacks."[11] Willis also suggested that genetic factors make the "weaker sex" more

prone to migraine, but this predisposition was shaped by "a sedentary life, full meals on an empty stomach, confined air and high
temperatures, disturbed sleep, anxious and prolonged study, un-
satisfied ambition, and perturbed passions."[12]

Like Willis, I have tried to discern what might precipitate or
aggravate my migraine attacks, particularly experimenting with my
diet and intake of various foods and beverages. I love coffee, and
caffeine withdrawal may trigger an attack of migraine.[13] I still am
not certain whether caffeine is good or bad for my migraine.
About 50 percent of people report that foods trigger their attacks.
Anything with monosodium glutamate (MSG) and strong cheese
containing tyramine have been most often incriminated.[14] The
evidence to support these claims is meager. My patients have also
identified a myriad of other precipitating events that may trigger
their attacks. Bright lights are the most common, but loud noises,
strong odors, and changes in the weather have often been suspect.
Many of the food and diet associations with migraine are purely
speculative. However, this has not stopped the plethora of junk-
science books on the subject. Many of these books promote diets
or other lifestyle advice for mitigating the migraine symptoms, but
precious few are based on actual research or documented evidence.

The increased prevalence of migraine in women suggests that
there are hormonal influences. In so-called menstrual migraine,
the attacks are synchronous with the menstrual cycle and disappear with the onset of menopause.[15] Menstrual migraine is usually
without aura, but the headaches last longer and are more likely to
relapse. The headaches typically occur just before menstruation
but may arise in the middle of the menstrual cycle, concurrent
with ovulation. Menstrual migraine usually remits during pregnancy. Unfortunately, to this day, the exact mechanism wherein female sex hormones, such as estrogen or progesterone, precipitate
or aggravate migraine is not clear.[16] In addition, the therapeutic
efficacy of hormone replacement therapy in preventing menstrual
migraine has been debated without a clear resolution.

Migraine, like every other chronic pain condition, is caused by a fusion of genetic and environmental factors. As with fibromyalgia, there is a strong genetic component to migraine, but no single candidate gene has been found, except in a rare form of migraine termed "familial hemiplegic migraine."[17] The genetic link is particularly evident in classic migraine with aura, which very often runs in families. It is likely that multiple genes interact with environmental factors to increase migraine susceptibility. Epigenetic factors, such as altered DNA methylation, enhance the susceptibility to migraine.[18]

Migraine is a central nervous system pain disorder. Sir William Gowers, in 1907, described migraine as a spreading neurologic phenomenon, commenting that "the process is very mysterious. There is a peculiar form of activity which seems to spread, like the ripples in the pond into which a stone is thrown, and in the regions through which the active ripple waves have passed, is left like molecular disturbance of the structure."[19] The author and superb neurologist Oliver Sacks described migraine as a "physical event which may also from the start, or later become, an emotional event. . . . [I]t is the prototype of a psychophysiological reaction."[20]

Until the 1970s, most scientists thought migraine to be a vascular phenomenon, with the pain related to excessive constriction and dilatation of cerebral blood vessels. It is now known that migraine is caused by alterations in nerve impulses in the brain, and any vascular changes are secondary reactions to pain.[21] This central nervous system brain reactivity was termed "cortical spreading depression," a self-propagating wave of electrical activity. The brain's visual cortex is responsible for the visual aura, while the headaches and the myriad of physical and emotional symptoms are the result of peripheral and central sensitization.[22] Brain imaging in migraine reveals altered structural and functional brain changes, including abnormal functional connectivity, similar to that in fibromyalgia.[23]

Not surprisingly, migraine is associated with generalized pain, including fibromyalgia, as well as sleep disturbances and mood disturbances. In one report, 70 percent of migraine subjects had fibromyalgia, compared to 26 percent with tension headaches.[24] Migraine patients are two to four times more likely to have comorbid major depression than healthy controls are.[25] Widespread heightened pain sensitivity is prominent in patients with migraine and correlates with headache frequency and severity, and with depression.[26]

Patients with migraine and fibromyalgia are often thought by family and health-care professionals to exaggerate their symptoms. George Beard observed that migraine patients, usually women, had difficulty persuading family, friends, and doctors about the seriousness of their conditions.[27] Similar to rheumatologists' disdain for fibromyalgia, many neurologists have been reluctant to treat migraine patients, although migraine has recently been more embraced by neurologists, particularly with new targeted therapies.

As in fibromyalgia, a better awareness and understanding of headaches emerged after experts got together to characterize and classify the various types of headaches, resulting in the *International Classification of Headache Disorders*.[28] Chronic migraine is diagnosed when the headaches occur on at least fifteen days per month for more than three months. My migraine would be classified as episodic. About 3 percent of people progress from episodic to chronic migraine each year. Fortunately, I am not one of them. Progression of episodic to chronic migraine correlates with increased central pain sensitivity.

What has set apart migraine from other chronic pain conditions has been the emergence of drugs targeted to putative neurochemical events—in other words, migraine-specific drugs. This has also promoted the claim that, in contrast to most chronic pain conditions, like fibromyalgia and chronic low back pain, migraine is a distinct neurologic disease with well-defined pathology.

Ergotamine was the first migraine-specific drug.[29] It was derived from ergot of rye, a crop disease caused by a fungus. Ergot extract had been used to stimulate uterine contractions and was thought to have vasoconstrictive effects. Since vasodilatation of cerebral blood vessels was the prevailing theory of migraine pathogenesis, ergotamine was tried in migraine and demonstrated some benefit. An ergot derivative, dihydroergotamine, a potent vasoconstrictor, is still used to treat acute migraine. The next drug used in migraine was methysergide, also derived from ergot.[30] It also stimulates serotonin neurotransmission. However, it caused significant toxicity and is no longer used.

In the 1990s triptans were introduced and demonstrated to be quite specific and effective for treating severe, acute migraine.[31] Triptans block brainstem pain pathways, targeting serotonin and hydroxytryptamine. Imitrex (sumatriptan) was the first triptan approved for use in the United States for migraine, in 1993. There are many currently available, and they can be given by injection, orally, and by nasal spray. They all work best when started at the first signs of a migraine attack. More recently, calcitonin gene-related peptide (CGRP), a potent vasodilator of cerebral blood vessels that also plays a role in neurotransmission, has been the target of migraine treatment.[32] Three drugs containing antibodies that target the CGRP receptor were the first medications developed explicitly to prevent migraine. They are each given by injection and have been quite effective in many patients for whom other treatments were ineffective.

The pathophysiology of acute migraine may differ from that of chronic migraine. As in fibromyalgia and chronic back and neck pain, central sensitization plays an important role when migraine is chronic. Therefore, chronic migraine treatment is often similar to that of fibromyalgia and includes analgesics, antidepressants—particularly amitriptyline—and various nonpharmacologic therapies. These include exercise, physical and cognitive therapies, and multiple therapeutic adjuncts, including acupuncture, various electrical and magnetic stimulation devices, and injection of various analgesics such as botulinum toxin (Botox).

Similar poor prognostic factors have been identified in migraine, tension headaches, and fibromyalgia. These include depression, anxiety, poor sleep, and poor coping mechanisms.[33] A century ago such psychosocial issues were considered the cause of migraine, as characterized by the title of Francis Graham Crookshank's 1926 book, *Migraine and Other Common Neuroses*.[34] He wrote, "The mind has the casting vote . . . and what we call the body is subordinate to it. The last word, the final choice is with our will."

Our current biopsychological illness model rejects such mind-over-matter advice. Migraine is best understood as a tapestry of interwoven genetic, biologic, and environmental factors. As each of these factors is better elucidated, treatment for migraine will continue to evolve.

MIGRAINE DIAGNOSIS

- Unilateral, throbbing headache
- Visual aura
- Multiple other physical and psychological symptoms, including fibromyalgia
- Worsening of symptoms with activity, bright lights
- Female predominance and hormonal influences

MIGRAINE TREATMENT

- Analgesics, anti-inflammatory medications
- Triptans, like Imitrex, for acute migraine attack
- Possible prevention of attacks through CRGP inhibitors
- Multimodal nonpharmacologic chronic pain management
- Avoidance of triggers (mainly individual since evidence is anecdotal)

7

TENSION HEADACHES; JAW AND FACIAL PAIN

Denise has had headaches all her life. These occur almost daily and are associated with neck, facial, and jaw pain. Most days she gets rid of the headache quickly by taking a few aspirin or ibuprofen and massaging her neck and shoulders. But she says that when she gets stressed or doesn't get a good night's sleep, the headaches can ruin her day. The headaches are usually bilateral and dull, and the muscles around her neck get tight and sore.

At age twenty Denise was evaluated by an oral surgeon, who found clicking when she opened her jaw widely. She had special X-rays and imaging studies and was told that she had a temporomandibular joint disorder, now called temporomandibular disorder (TMD). Denise wore an appliance at night for a few months without any improvement and then had surgery to correct jaw malalignment. The surgery did not help her headaches, and her facial pain worsened.

When I met Denise, she was age thirty-eight and most bothered by her daily headaches and the associated neck, facial, and upper back pain. She told me that at its worst "it feels like a tight band is compressing my head and a heavy weight is on my neck and shoulders." She also complained of lower back pain, poor sleep, and fatigue. Her examination was notable for tenderness and spasm throughout the muscle around her head and neck, especially at the jaw and temple.

Denise's headaches fit the pattern of muscle or tension-type headaches. Tension-type headaches are ubiquitous, occurring in more than 85 percent of the population.[1] For most of us, tension headaches are more of a nuisance, neither severe nor long-lasting. In contrast to migraine and fibromyalgia, there is no good evidence for a genetic link; they are not associated with an array of other physical symptoms, may not require medical therapy, and seldom cause long-term disability. Unlike in Denise's case, the vast majority of tension headaches are episodic rather than daily.

The term *tension headache* implies that these headaches are a result of emotional stress and that muscle tension or spasm is the source of pain. Studies have found no greater levels of stress or mood disturbances in tension headaches than in migraine or any other chronic pain disorder. As with the vascular theory of migraine, the muscle tension theory has been largely debunked. Peripheral muscle spasm and tenderness are often present and may be associated with what are called "myofascial trigger points."[2] John F. Kennedy, who had chronic migraine and tension headaches as well as chronic low back pain, was treated with frequent myofascial trigger point injections by Dr. Janet Travell, a physical medicine and rehabilitation specialist. She and many of her disciples believed that these trigger points were areas of distinct muscle pathology that caused the pain. Indeed, these myofascial trigger points may respond to massage, stretching, or local injections of anesthetic agents. However, myofascial trigger points represent a physiologic reaction to pain and are not discrete areas of muscle inflammation. They are not the root cause of headaches but the result of chronic pain, just like the tender points so prominent in fibromyalgia.

Chronic tension headaches, such as Denise had, are caused by central nervous system sensitization, just as fibromyalgia is. There is experimental evidence of generalized pain hypersensitivity and altered response to various stimuli in the brain and spinal cord.[3] In a population study, there was a strong correlation of altered pain perception with development of chronic headaches, best explained by central sensitization.[4]

Denise's headaches and facial pain were attributed to TMD although, in hindsight, she did not meet the current criteria for that disorder. Her unsuccessful jaw surgery was the all too familiar plight of countless patients until TMD was better defined and its natural history better understood. For years TMD was erroneously thought to be caused by a structural abnormality of the jaw joint. Temporomandibular joint pain (TMJ) was the name given by dentists based on the biomedical disease model that the symptoms were attributed to dental malocclusions. Indeed, jaw arthritis, not rare in rheumatoid arthritis, can cause severe orofacial pain and headaches, and malalignment between the upper and lower jaw is a factor in some patients with TMD. But dental malocclusions or other anatomic issues are only part of the usual biopsychological puzzle of TMD, which includes genetic, environmental, and psychological factors.

About one in four of us will have episodes of chronic orofacial pain, and 5 percent of the population report chronic pain in the jaw with chronic headaches and facial pain.[5] Women are affected more than men, and TMD often begins in early adulthood. The annual cost of TMD management in the United States is $4 billion.[6] Most commonly, dentists are the first health-care professionals to see people with TMD symptoms.

TMD represents a heterogenous group of head and neck pains that may or may not include jaw pathology and encompass various diagnoses, such as myofascial pain, myalgias, and arthralgias of the head and neck, with referred headaches as well as TMJ joint disease or dysfunction. Diagnosis of TMD related to joint or muscle pain without anatomic jaw abnormalities includes pain in the jaw, temple, and ear, modified by jaw movement and often with headache in the temple region.[7] Confirming a diagnosis of TMD associated with structural jaw abnormalities requires symptoms such as clicking, popping, or locking; limited jaw movement with pain, and abnormalities on palpation of the jaw.[8] This requires an evaluation with a dentist or oral surgeon and may include special X-rays and imaging studies of the affected jaw.

Other causes of orofacial pain must be excluded. These include migraine, already discussed, and trigeminal neuralgia, to be discussed in the chapter on neuropathic pain. Most often a neurologist will be the best specialist to help to differentiate such disorders from TMD.

TMD was one of the first chronic pain conditions found to have a strong genetic influence, including an association with the gene that controls catechol-O-methyltransferase (COMT) expression.[9] TMD is also associated with behavioral and psychological factors, including sleep disturbances, depression, and catastrophizing. Like fibromyalgia, it fits best into a biopsychological illness framework with central sensitization as the driving force behind its pain chronicity. Brain neuroimaging has shown functional and structural changes in the thalamus and prefrontal cortex in TMD.[10] In various reports, between 25 and 70 percent of patients with TMD also have fibromyalgia.[11]

The first goal in treating TMD is to determine whether there is associated structural jaw pathology with referral to an oral specialist. If this is found, patient education regarding jaw movements; avoidance of clenching, teeth grinding (bruxism), and chewing gum and hard foods; and dietary approaches are important. Massage, various compresses, and physical therapy, with specific jaw exercises, are routine. Oral appliances that reduce jaw movement and redistribute bite forces are the next step, and if all that fails, jaw injections with anesthetics or corticosteroids are usually recommended. In contrast to twenty years ago, when Denise had unsuccessful surgery, TMJ surgery is now reserved for patients with documented anatomic abnormalities and persistent severe jaw pain despite nonsurgical management. There is little evidence that surgery improves the outcome in the vast majority of patients with TMD.[12]

Every patient with TMD should be managed with the same multidisciplinary program outlined for fibromyalgia and for chronic headaches. Often this will be initiated in primary care but may include specialists, particularly a neurologist if chronic tension headaches are the primary concern. Treatment includes medications and nonpharmacologic therapy. There is limited evidence for the effectiveness of NSAIDs; local anesthetics; antidepressants, like amitriptyline; anticonvulsants, such as gabapentin; and botulinum toxin injections.[13] Soft-tissue or so-called myofascial injections have been helpful for the localized neck and upper torso pain and can relieve tension headaches.[14] Cognitive behavioral treatment (CBT) or other mindfulness training has been found to be effective in the treatment of TMD.[15]

DIAGNOSIS OF TENSION HEADACHE AND JAW AND FACIAL PAIN

- Tension headaches, the most common type of headache, are usually mild to moderate, bilateral, and associated with muscle tenderness in the neck and shoulders.
- There is a strong association of tension headaches with temporomandibular disorder (TMD).
- TMD may or may not be associated with anatomic jaw problems.
- The symptoms of TMD include pain in the jaw, temple, and ear, modified by jaw movement, often with headache in the temple region.
- Jaw clicking and locking should prompt a careful dental examination.

TREATMENT OF TENSION HEADACHES AND JAW AND FACIAL PAIN

- If jaw pathology is found, oral manual education, appliances, and localized therapy are helpful.
- Jaw surgery is now considered to be a last resort in patients with well-documented anatomic abnormalities.

- Management of tension headache and TMD follows the multi-disciplinary, biopsychological model, including pharmacologic and nonpharmacologic therapy.

8

CHRONIC LOW BACK AND NECK PAIN; THE ROLE OF TRAUMA AND INJURY

Frida Kahlo (1907–1954), one of the most famous artists of the twentieth century, suffered from a lifetime of chronic pain following a series of illnesses and trauma. At age six, she came down with polio and spent nine months in bed, which resulted in severe right leg pain, muscle atrophy, and weakness.[1] She also experienced generalized pain and chronic fatigue, which today might have been diagnosed as fibromyalgia or postpolio syndrome.

She overcame this early illness and was accepted to the finest educational institute in Mexico, Escuela Nacional Preparatoria, as one of thirty-five girls in a school of two thousand students. Tragically, on her way home from school, her bus was crushed by a streetcar. She suffered fractures of the clavicle, ribs, spine, pelvis, and elbow, and both ankles and shoulders were dislocated. A metal rod punctured her abdomen. It was a miracle that she survived, but she was left with severe, chronic pain.

Kahlo had unrelenting lower back pain, felt to be caused by a congenital scoliosis and the severe back injury and spinal fractures. She went through a number of failed back operations and in 1950 had a spinal fusion of the lower four lumbar vertebrae. I had that operation about ten years ago and was one of the fortunate ones who got great results with significant reduction in my back pain and sciatica. Unfortunately, Kahlo's surgery was a failure. Kahlo's personal life was riddled with events that are risk factors for chronic pain. She was sexually abused as a child; had a history of depression, drug, and alcohol abuse; and was embroiled in an abusive marriage with painter Diego Rivera.[2]

Kahlo had not only unremitting back pain but also severe stabbing pain throughout her body as well as physical and mental exhaustion. In her striking self-portrait, *The Broken Column*, Kahlo's spinal column is replaced by large metal rods, and her body is bound together by a leather corset.[3] Large nails pierce through multiple points on her face, neck, shoulders, trunk, and pelvis. Some of my rheumatology colleagues in Mexico have surmised that Kahlo had post-traumatic fibromyalgia, and the nails represent locations of the multiple tender points characteristic of fibromyalgia.[4]

Kahlo and her physicians attributed her chronic back pain to the injuries and physical trauma she suffered at age seventeen. For centuries, the public and the medical profession have assumed that back pain is primarily a structural disorder. The more severe the injury, the more out of alignment the back vertebrae, the more unrelenting will be the pain. It then followed that getting rid of back pain would require identifying the structural cause and removing it or fixing it.

More than 80 percent of adults will experience low back pain during their lifetime.[5] In any three-month period, approximately 30 percent of adults report low back pain, and 15 percent report headaches and neck pain.[6] For most individuals, the pain is self-limited, lasting from days to weeks. However, at least 10 percent of the population will suffer from chronic low back pain that lasts more than three months at a time. Following the usual biomedical disease model, doctors used to assume that if we looked hard enough, we could always pinpoint some anatomic anomaly for the pain. We have now learned that a structural abnormality in the spine is found in less than 10 percent of cases of chronic low back pain.[7]

There are some life-threatening causes of low back pain, such as cancer, spinal infection, or spinal cord compression, that usually begin abruptly with associated symptoms, such as fever, weight loss, or incapacitating neurologic signs. These are typically diagnosed quickly and are always a medical emergency. Less than 1 percent of patients with acute back pain seen in primary care will have a life-threatening cause for their pain.

Then there are more common but less serious structural causes of low back pain, such as vertebral disk degeneration or spinal stenosis. With sensitive radiologic techniques such as MRI, these potential structural causes of back pain are nowadays picked up frequently. However, they are often incidental findings and not necessarily the source of the pain. Most often, failed back surgery has been the result of an overly simplistic, mechanistic approach to chronic pain and the poor correlation of anatomic abnormalities with symptoms.

In the 1990s back surgery was often recommended for patients with protruded lumbar discs on MRI until it was found that 20 to 60 percent of adults with no back pain had evidence of some disc herniations on imaging studies.[8] Finding protruded lumbar discs or some narrowing between the lower lumbar vertebrae is commonplace and does not correlate with chronic low back pain. Back imaging should not be routinely ordered in people with low back pain but reserved for patients with worrisome symptoms or prior to any surgical consideration.[9] Removal of a herniated disk is no longer considered in patients with chronic back pain unless there are associated neurologic symptoms or the patients have failed to improve after nonsurgical therapy.

Despite the poor correlation of imaging abnormalities in the lumbar spine with chronic back pain, there has been a 300 percent increase in lumbar MRIs and a 220 percent increase in spinal fusion rates in the past ten years.[10] As in cases of excess surgery for lumbar disc herniation, many patients with back pain and spinal stenosis may not respond well to surgery. At least one out of five people who have lumbar fusion surgery will have persistent back pain.[11] After my chronic back pain kept increasing and interfering more with my life, I elected to have a surgical lumbar fusion. Even after my back surgeon showed me the MRIs demonstrating increasing vertebral bone deterioration and degeneration, I knew that the decision to undergo the lumbar fusion was hardly straightforward. I had been faithful with my back rehabilitation and physical therapy program for two years but was still having a lot of back pain. After consulting with two back surgeons, I did opt for surgery. Even when chronic back pain can be conclusively attributed to structural degeneration in the spine, that can't always be surgically alleviated.

What the public fails to realize is that for the vast majority of people with chronic back pain, there are no defined bone, nerve, or joint abnormalities. This is often labeled as "nonspecific" back pain. Chronic, nonspecific low back pain is the most common cause of work-related disability. Certain medical professionals, particularly chiropractors and physical therapists, often attribute the pain to physical events, such as muscle spasm or vertebral misalignment. There is scant evidence to back up these assertions.

Since most of us will have some disc protrusion or degenerative arthritic findings in our back by the time we are fifty, it is always tempting to attribute our pain to these physical changes. It certainly was reasonable to think that Frida Kahlo's chronic back pain was caused by the spinal damage following the bus crash and that back surgery might improve her pain. However, after nearly a century of failed back surgeries, physicians now better appreciate that chronic back pain usually cannot be attributed to an injury or structural abnormality.

Psychosocial factors are as important in chronic low back pain as in every chronic pain condition we are discussing. For example, pain severity and subsequent disability was worse in chronic back pain patients who retained an attorney, initiated litigation, or filed for workers' compensation than in those who did not.[12] Personal beliefs about back pain have profound influences on pain severity and chronicity. In a study of 2,400 Canadians, one-third had experienced back pain lasting for more than one week.[13] The vast majority of people held a pessimistic view of back pain and thought the chronic low back pain would eventually stop them from working. Those who took time off from work and considered that bed rest was important to their recovery had more persistent pain.

Until about ten years ago, back pain was treated like an injury, typically with prolonged bed rest. It makes sense that strenuous work or unusual exercise might cause chronic low back pain. However, the majority of studies have found that psychosocial factors are more important than physical factors in predicting who will develop chronic back pain, even in workers with physically demanding jobs.[14]

Even when an injury or physical trauma has triggered the back pain, the likelihood of an individual developing chronic pain does not correlate with that initial event. Attributing the persistent back pain to an injury that should have healed long ago interferes with recovery.

Pain chronicity is linked to central sensitization. One out of three women with chronic low back pain also report widespread pain consistent with fibromyalgia, and those with widespread pain have greater mood disturbances and are more often on disability.[15] Brain imaging abnormalities in patients with chronic low back pain are similar to those in fibromyalgia, including gray matter loss and alterations in regional brain connectivity.[16]

We have learned the same lessons from chronic neck pain. Here, too, there is little correlation of anatomic or structural changes with symptoms. As mentioned, the prevalence of chronic neck pain is similar to that of chronic back pain, occurring in 10 to 20 percent of adults. As with low back pain, there are rare life-threatening causes of neck pain, but typically these present acutely and are always medical emergencies. And, as in low back pain, occasionally neurologic or degenerative cervical abnormalities will be the cause of the neck pain. But most often this is not the case.

Despite the absence of a defined anatomic explanation, chronic neck pain has been closely linked to physical trauma, fostered by "whiplash," a term initially coined by Harold Crowe in 1928 to

describe an acceleration-deceleration neck injury following a motor vehicle accident.[17] Whiplash injury subsequently was expanded to include any form of neck trauma causing chronic neck
and upper extremity pain with no obvious anatomic source. A
Quebec task force proposed that "rather than trying to view whiplash as a specific, anatomically definable injury, this diverse cluster
of post-whiplash symptoms be reconceptualized as forming a 'general illness' with widespread symptom presentation—that is, an
illness in which symptoms arise from and are modulated by pathology, psychological responses and social context."[18]

Symptoms of chronic whiplash beyond the requisite neck pain
include low back pain, mood disturbances, sleep disturbances,
cognitive disturbances, dizziness, and numbness and tingling in
the arms and legs, all signs suggestive of central sensitization.
Brain imaging has revealed decreased regional gray matter volume, similar to that described in fibromyalgia.[19]

Fifty percent of patients with whiplash will end up in chronic
pain and on long-term disability.[20] Collision factors, such as speed
of the car, site of the impact, or damage to the vehicle did not
correlate with chronic pain or functional incapacity. The factors
that correlated best with poor outcome and long-term disability
included prior history of chronic pain and depression, and psychosocial factors such as postinjury anxiety and catastrophizing and
seeking compensation and litigation.[21]

We have all experienced pain after lifting heavy objects or per-
forming some manual labor for the first time. Fortunately, that
pain is generally short-lived. It is tempting to link physical trauma
or injury to chronic pain even without sound medical evidence.
The term *whiplash* suggests that the chronic pain was the result of
the car accident or other neck trauma. This hypothetical, causal
explanation has promoted a series of personal reactions, including
blame, anger, rumination, and a sense of helplessness. On a societal level, medical-legal uncertainty around injury litigation may
interfere with individual patient recovery.

In the 1980s thousands of medical claims for nonspecific neck
and arm pain attributed to various workplace injuries were filed in

Australia.[22] This was termed repetitive strain injury (RSI) and began in electrical process workers but quickly involved many jobs requiring repetitive hand/arm use. Recognizable pain conditions such as carpal tunnel syndrome, tendinitis, or epicondylitis were excluded in every instance, and no specific pathology was found. Between 1980, when the term RSI was popularized in the press, and 1985, the insurance claims for such injuries increased in New South Wales by 1,200 percent.[23] Millions of dollars were spent on redesigning workstations despite no evidence that physical trauma was the source of pain. As soon as the government stopped paying out claims for work-related injury, the RSI epidemic faded away. In retrospect RSI was an example of sociopolitical forces merging to greatly change people's perception and reaction to a potential cause of their suffering. An Australian rheumatologist stated, "Despite intensive litigation, compensation and publicity . . . most persons are now back at work . . . doing the same activity and using the same equipment. . . . In Australia persons who have had 'RSI' now seldom talk of it."[24]

There are many other instances where social policies and economic factors have far outweighed putative biologic causes in perpetuating chronic pain. In Norway in the 1990s there was an "explosion of chronic-whiplash cases . . . people are claiming compensation from mechanical forces not more than you would get in daily life, from coughing, sneezing, running down the steps, plopping into a chair. And they are getting millions of kroner in compensation. It's mass hysteria."[25] Shortly after the Norwegian spike in whiplash cases, a research study about chronic pain in the aftermath of a motor vehicle accident was done in Lithuania.[26] In that country there was little awareness of whiplash and no personal injury insurance. The investigators there compared people involved in car accidents to age- and sex-matched people from the same town with no history of a car accident. In Lithuania the incidence of chronic neck pain was the same in both groups.

As with fibromyalgia, chronic back and neck pain are best understood with a biopsychological illness model. Although my rheumatology colleagues from Mexico postulate that Frida Kahlo suffered from "post-traumatic fibromyalgia," most of us in the field no longer use the term *post-traumatic*. Physical trauma is just one of many factors that people attribute to the onset of their pain and suffering. Individuals who believe their fibromyalgia began after physical trauma don't differ clinically from other patients with fibromyalgia, except for having a worse outcome. People especially vulnerable to central sensitization, like Kahlo was, are the ones most likely to experience chronic pain following a minor or major traumatic event. Individual factors, such as previous chronic pain, a history of mood disturbances, and poor coping mechanisms such as catastrophizing and avoidance behavior, are more important than biologic or physical factors in predicting if postinjury pain will become chronic.

The model of injury causing pain led to the unfortunate "rest" recipe for treating chronic neck and back pain. Until ten years ago, complete bed rest for up to a week was standard management for low back pain. That, we now understand, was the worst possible approach; we now know that the quicker we can get people moving, the better. As we will discuss, level of physical fitness is a major determinant of who will develop chronic low back pain. Both physical and psychological workplace factors contribute to low back pain. We are aware that heavy lifting or working with arms often over our heads will increase back and neck pain, and we usually pay attention to such physical dynamics. We may be less aware of the influence of job satisfaction and social engagement in our chronic pain. Improving the outcome of chronic low back and neck pain will necessitate turning away from the injury/ physical damage approach to individualized mind and body management.

IMPORTANT POINTS ABOUT NECK AND BACK PAIN AND TRAUMA

- Chronic back and neck pain are most often not caused by structural abnormalities in the cervical or lumbar spine.

- Imaging studies, such as MRI, often demonstrate such anatomic changes, but these may not correlate with chronic pain.
- Such discrepancies, so-called false positive test results, may lead to unnecessary procedures and failed back or neck surgery.
- Surgery or invasive procedures for chronic back or neck pain may be effective in patients who have failed a more conservative approach and should be decided upon after consulting appropriate specialists.
- Treatment for chronic neck and back pain should include attention to physical factors, such as posture and exercise, and psychological factors, including in the home and workplace.

9

COMPLEX REGIONAL PAIN AND NEUROPATHIC PAIN

Becky was a healthy, athletic young women until she fell at work and badly injured her right wrist and hand. X-rays did not reveal a fracture, and her right wrist was placed in a splint. The pain intensified over the next few weeks. She saw an orthopedic hand specialist, and further tests, including an MRI of the wrist and hand, were performed but were unrevealing. The wrist was then put in a cast, but soon her whole forearm began to ache and swell.

When the cast was removed after a few more weeks, Becky said, "My whole right forearm looked blue and it was swollen. The pain was intense and burning, radiating up to my upper arm." The hand specialist suspected that Becky was developing complex regional pain syndrome (CRPS) and gave her opioids for pain relief. Becky also began a course of physical therapy, including deep tissue massage, alternating heat and cold applications, and movement treatment. But every time Becky tried to move her right hand or arm, the pain worsened. A two-week trial of prednisone, a corticosteroid, did not help. After six months she was appalled and said, "My arm looked withered, and it had lost all its color and hair. My fingernails were falling out. The slightest touch killed me, especially if anything cold or hot even brushed against my skin."

She then saw a neurologist who confirmed the diagnosis of CRPS. The doctor increased the opioids and added gabapentin, but the pain did not get better. Over the next year Becky was treated with various injections, including different anesthetics, a sympathetic ganglion block, and an implantable nerve stimulator, and she received an infusion of immunoglobulin, all to no avail.

When I met Becky, her pain had been going on for more than three years. She was tearful and seemed very apprehensive. Becky had never been able to go back to work and could barely function independently at home. She described a bed-to-chair existence at home and became very depressed, admitting to thoughts of suicide. Her right arm was atrophied and pale-looking, and her fingers were contracted in a fist. It was difficult to pry them open. The extremity felt cooler than the opposite arm. She had very little range of motion of that elbow and shoulder. The right hand and arm were extremely tender to any touch.

CRPS was described in the sixteenth century by Ambroise Paré. Paré, a surgeon and barber, reported that his patients would sometimes get severe, chronic pain after being treated with a phlebotomy, "bloodletting," in an arm.[1] In 1864 the neurologist Silas Weir Mitchell reported that a number of Civil War gunshot victims developed persistent burning pain with shiny, red skin in the extremity that was shot. He coined the term "causalgia," from a Greek word meaning heat and pain. In 1946 James Evans, a Massachusetts physician, suggested that the symptoms were caused by aberrations in the sympathetic nervous system and changed the name to "reflex sympathetic dystrophy."[2] During the twentieth century more than two hundred names were given to this condition.[3] With little evidence that the sympathetic nervous system was at fault, the name was changed to its current one, complex regional pain syndrome (CRPS), in 1994.[4] This descriptive term implied that the pathophysiology was unknown.

As in Becky's case, CRPS most often follows trauma to an extremity. This includes fractures, sprains, or crush injuries. It also may develop after immobility of an extremity, such as wearing a cast or an arm sling. Even having an intravenous line or having chest pain for a few days may lead to CRPS. Type I CRPS occurs in the absence of nerve injury, and Type II occurs after a nerve injury, although nerve conduction studies have not found any consistent differences in Type I or Type II CRPS.[5] CRPS is three or four times more common in women, with a peak age range of forty to sixty.[6]

Diagnosis of CRPS is based on the symptoms of regional pain in an extremity, usually following some traumatic event. The pain is usually intense and persists long after the injury. There are sensory changes, such as Becky's hypersensitivity to touch and heat or cold; skin changes, including color or temperature changes; and anatomic changes, such as her arm atrophy and loss of motion. There are no diagnostic laboratory or X-ray findings, but a bone scan after a few months of symptoms will often reveal a patchy osteoporosis (active bone resorption).

Is CRPS a neuropathic pain disorder? Neuropathic pain is the result of injury- or disease-related damage to peripheral nerves. Classic examples include diabetic neuropathy and postherpetic neuralgia (shingles). In these situations, the pain follows the sensory distribution of the affected nerve and is of a burning or shock-like quality. There is a loss of sensation in that nerve, which can be documented by physical testing or by nerve conduction velocity tests, including an electromyogram (EMG).

Diabetic neuropathy is the most common cause of neuropathic pain and best fits the biomedical model of peripheral nerve damage causing the pain. About 25 percent of patients with diabetes develop neuropathic pain.[7] The degree of peripheral nerve damage plays a role in who gets pain and who doesn't, but it is not the only factor. Female gender, genetic predisposition, and central nervous system pain processing are also involved. Neuroimaging has found clear differences in the brains of patients with painful compared to painless diabetic neuropathy. These include increased reactivity in pain-regulating areas such as the anterior insula, the thalamus, and the somatosensory cortex.[8]

Trigeminal neuralgia is also classified as neuropathic pain. It causes electric, burning, episodic pain in the fifth (trigeminal) cranial nerve. The pain usually lasts for seconds to a minute but can be very severe. There are often facial muscle spasms, which gave rise to the old term "tic douloureux." It also may cause headaches, eye tearing, and nasal congestion. Trigeminal neuralgia is usually caused by compression of the nerve from nearby aberrant arteries or veins. Sometimes, surgical decompression is necessary to relieve pressure on the trigeminal nerve. Although trigeminal neuralgia is classified as neuropathic pain, central nervous system mechanisms play an important role. Structural and functional changes, including gray matter loss in the thalamus and abnormal connectivity between pain-transmitting areas of the brain, are present in patients with trigeminal neuralgia.[9]

Patients with neuropathic pain also suffer from chronic and widespread pain, sleep disturbances, and mood disturbances.[10] Since central pain plays a role in all forms of chronic pain, is there any rationale to classify pain as neuropathic? If neuropathic pain is caused solely by direct nerve injury, identifying and removing the physical cause of that injury might cure the condition. Getting blood sugar under optimal control should improve the outcome of diabetic neuropathy. Antiviral therapy might lessen the severity of zoster neuropathy. Removing the anatomic compression of the fifth cranial nerve could cure trigeminal neuropathy. However, these treatments are only effective in the early stages of neuropathic pain. Once the pain becomes chronic, central sensitization drives the pain.

Identifying pain as neuropathic would matter if treatment varied based on that pain classification. For example, neuropathic pain responds best to antiseizure medications such as carbamazepine or gabapentin. Those medications also can be effective in fibromyalgia, a central pain disorder. There is limited evidence for immune activation in neuropathic pain, and various types of immune therapy have been advocated. This was the rationale for Becky to have received intravenous immunoglobulin for the treatment of her CRPS. However, CRPS, neuropathic pain, and fibromyalgia are not classic immune diseases such as rheumatoid arthritis or systemic lupus erythematosus.

Since the burning pain and skin changes in CRPS do not follow any sensory nerve distribution and nerve velocity studies are normal, CRPS is not classified as a neuropathic pain condition. In general, classifying pain as structural/inflammatory, neuropathic, or central is misleading, since all chronic pain has peripheral and central elements. When any pain becomes chronic, central mechanisms become dominant. We can't ignore possible peripheral factors, but treatment must focus on pain hypersensitivity.

The pathophysiology behind CRPS, as well as each of the chronic pain disorders, fits best in a mind *and* body framework. Multidisciplinary team management is considered to be the treatment of choice for CRPS and neuropathic pain, just as it is for fibromyalgia or chronic low back pain. In CRPS, physical trauma or injury is clearly an inciting event. However, it can be quite trivial. Fibromyalgia patients and those with chronic back and neck pain also often attribute the onset of symptoms to trauma or physical injury. The common denominator seems to be loss of movement, in some people just for a few days. Becky's prolonged arm immobility, not the severity of the wrist sprain, was the key physical trigger. Stopping activity and exercise when suffering from fibromyalgia or a week of bed rest when having low back pain results in prolonged pain. Patients with post-traumatic stress disorder (PTSD) are more prone to CRPS.[11] The severity of CRPS correlates with a patient's level of anxiety, particularly about long-term disability.[12]

Becky had been treated aggressively for her severe pain with the latest technologies, including sympathetic nerve block and implant of a spinal cord stimulator, with little effect on her pain. Although there is little evidence that CRPS is an immune disease, Becky was also given multiple intravenous infusions of immunoglobulin, with no benefit. She had become frustrated and felt increasingly hopeless.

The depth of her depression had not been recognized until she admitted to suicidal thoughts. Suicide risk is much greater in patients with chronic pain than in the general population. As discussed in chapter 2, depression is present in the majority of patients with chronic pain and the more intractable the pain, the greater the depression, increasing the risk for suicide.

Suicidality is more related to psychosocial than physical factors. The most important risk factor for suicidality in chronic pain patients was found to be unemployment or disability.[13] General risk factors for depression, not specific for suicidality, include anger, poor sleep, smoking, alcohol use, catastrophizing, and hopelessness. Opioids, which Becky had been taking for three years, increase the risk for suicide, and 40 percent of suicides involve opioids.[14] Suicide prevention intervention should be included in chronic pain management programs.

Our mental health professional used a combination of antidepressant medications, individual counseling, and cognitive behavioral therapy to counter Becky's sense of hopelessness and major depression. She was slowly weaned off opioids; she continued on gabapentin, and duloxetine was added. A physical medicine and rehabilitation specialist and physical therapist began intense rehabilitation, which included graded motor imagery, a program using visual cues, thermal biofeedback, and mirror images to get the affected arm moving. Becky made great progress with an aquatic exercise program.

She slowly but gradually felt much more hopeful, noting, "It felt so good to be able to move again and be active." The range of motion of her hand and arm gradually improved, as did the muscle atrophy. After about six months she was able to return to work as an elementary school teacher.

SYMPTOMS AND IMPORTANT POINTS ABOUT CRPS AND NEUROPATHIC PAIN

- Chronic regional pain syndrome (CRPS) usually follows trauma to an extremity.
- It is associated with sensory, skin, and anatomic abnormalities.
- Immobility is an important physical initiating event in CRPS.

- Neuropathic pain generally implies direct nerve injury, but the central nervous system is a major contributor to the chronicity and severity of pain.
- CRPS and most chronic pain conditions follow the mind *and* body model and should be treated with an integrated multidisciplinary team.

10

CHRONIC BOWEL, BLADDER, AND PELVIC PAIN

Susan was referred to me by her gastroenterologist. She was a healthy-appearing forty-year-old woman who about 10 years earlier had been diagnosed with irritable bowel syndrome (IBS) by the gastroenterologist. She told me, "I have had a sensitive stomach all my life." At age twelve she began having bouts of cramping lower abdominal pain and diarrhea. She was thought to be intolerant of gluten although blood tests were not consistent with celiac disease. She tried to avoid dietary gluten, but it did not make much difference in her symptoms.

Over the next ten years, Susan continued to have these gastrointestinal symptoms, at times so severe that she would miss a day or two of school. She restricted what she ate and was always quite thin. One of her doctors suspected that she had an eating disorder. Another diagnosed her with multiple food allergies. The gastroenterologist did a thorough examination, including multiple blood tests and a colonoscopy, all of which were normal. He concluded that she had IBS. With further dietary advice and reassurance that there was no progressive gastrointestinal disease, Susan's symptoms improved.

Shortly after the birth of her second child, Susan began having intense pelvic pain, most prominent just before each menstrual cycle. Her gynecologist found diffuse vulvar tenderness but no other abnormalities. Inserting a tampon or having intercourse greatly aggravated the pain. Susan did have a history of frequent bladder infections, including two that were both knocked out quickly with antibiotics during her pregnancy. Now there was no evidence for a bladder or vaginal infection.

She consulted with a urologist, who performed a bladder ultrasound and cystoscopy, which were normal. Both her bladder function and structure were fine. He concluded that she most likely had interstitial cystitis. Around that time Susan also began noting generalized muscle pain and soreness as well as excess fatigue. Those symptoms prompted the referral to me. Her history and physical examination demonstrated that Susan had fibromyalgia.

Chronic bowel, bladder, and pelvic pain affect 10 to 30 percent of the population and most often is not caused by any defined organ pathology. It is important that any person with these symptoms undergo an appropriate examination, since infection, anatomic abnormalities, or a tumor could be the cause of such complaints. Susan was checked to be certain she did not have an infection or any disease that could cause her gastrointestinal and bladder symptoms. If initial testing does not demonstrate any physical cause of bowel, bladder, and pelvic pain, none will likely be found. The gastrointestinal symptoms are labeled as irritable bowel syndrome (IBS). The genitourinary symptoms are labeled as interstitial cystitis, pelvic/bladder pain syndrome, or urologic chronic pelvic pain syndrome (UCPPS). IBS and UCPPS are sometimes bunched under the title of functional pain disorders, implying that there is no internal organ dysfunction. These functional pain disorders overlap with each other and with fibromyalgia.

IRRITABLE BOWEL SYNDROME (IBS)

Approximately 10 to 15 percent of people will meet criteria for IBS at some point, and IBS makes up 25 to 50 percent of referrals to gastroenterologists in the United States.[1] It is twice as common in women, with a peak age from thirty to fifty. IBS is diagnosed based on symptoms and the exclusion of an inflammatory gastrointestinal disease, such as ulcerative colitis or Crohn's disease. IBS is subdivided into diarrhea- or constipation-predominant. Symptoms include cramping abdominal pain, bloating, and either constipation or diarrhea. The physical and laboratory examinations are unremarkable, and in selected cases a colonoscopy will be done to exclude any intestinal pathology. Symptoms often wax and wane but, as with Susan, they tend to be chronic. Stress and certain foods, particularly heavy meals, often aggravate the symptoms.

IBS is caused by alterations in gut motility triggered by gastrointestinal and central nervous system hyperirritability. There is some evidence of gut immune activation and inflammation, and there is a role for infectious agents such as altered fecal microflora. IBS sometimes follows a bacterial or viral gastroenteritis and also may be triggered by food sensitivity. Whatever the initiating events in IBS, the central nervous system hypersensitivity perpetuates the chronic pain. This has been referred to as the "gut-brain axis." We are each aware of this interaction when our stomachs get queasy or we need to rush to the toilet while in a stressful situation.

Research in IBS has demonstrated strikingly similar findings to that in fibromyalgia. Not surprisingly, 30 to 60 percent of patients with IBS, like Susan, also suffer from fibromyalgia.[2] There is some hereditary influence on IBS. Environmental risk factors include a history of mood disorders and childhood stress, most notably sexual or physical abuse. Susan did report a history of such abuse in childhood. There is evidence of generalized pain hypersensitivity to multiple stimuli. Brain imaging has shown structural and functional changes in regions that are key to pain transmission.[3] These areas of altered brain activity are most striking in brain areas that account for the emotional components of pain.

IBS symptoms often improve with simple dietary modification, especially if the person can identify offending foods. Excluding gas-forming foods, gluten, or lactose may help. IBS with constipation is treated first with soluble fiber or polyethylene glycol. If that fails, most gastroenterologists prescribe a medication such as Amitiza (lubiprostone) or Linzess (linaclotide), which increase intestinal fluid secretion. In IBS with diarrhea, Imodium (loperamide) has been most often prescribed. Amitriptyline, as used in fibromyalgia, can be quite effective in diarrhea-predominant IBS. Lotronex (alosetron) is approved for use in patients with severe diarrhea-predominant IBS. As with any chronic pain, management should include exercise, behavior modification, stress reduction, and, when necessary, antidepressants. Increased physical activity consisting of thirty to sixty minutes of moderate to vigorous exercise three times weekly was seen to result in improved IBS symptoms compared to control patients.[4]

CHRONIC BLADDER AND PELVIC PAIN

Chronic bladder and pelvic pain so often occur together that they are now classified jointly under the new diagnostic label "urologic chronic pelvic pain syndrome" (UCPPS).[5] In the past, pelvic pain was often termed "vulvodynia," erroneously suggesting that the pain was confined to the vulva. Between 5 and 10 percent of women report chronic vulvar pain that can't be traced to any anatomic abnormality or infection.[6] Most often the pain is not confined to the vulva but involves the pelvic region. As Susan described it, the pain is often aggravated by intercourse or any other pressure. Chronic bladder pain, particularly in women, was termed "interstitial cystitis," the diagnosis that Susan was given. This term was also misleading and the result of urologists' claim that bladder inflammation was causing the pain. This led to unsuccessful bladder instillation of various chemicals, such as dimethyl sulfoxide (DMSO). Research has revealed no evidence of bladder inflammation. Men with UCPPS may be diagnosed with chronic prostatitis, although prostatitis usually refers to bladder symptoms related to anatomic changes, such as benign prostatic hypertrophy.

Every patient with these bladder symptoms should have a urinalysis to exclude bladder or kidney infection and to determine if there is blood in the urine. Manual pelvic and prostate examinations are needed to exclude any anatomic lesions. If there is possible infection, tumor, or systemic disease, a urologist should be consulted and generally a bladder ultrasound and cystoscopy are performed.

Between 3 and 7 percent of women in the United States meet the new diagnostic criteria for UCPPS. The symptoms include chronic pain in the pelvis, urogenital region, or external genitalia with lower urinary symptoms such as urgency, frequency, and burning. Often patients have an inability to completely empty the bladder, needing to sit on the toilet for a long time to allow the urine to dribble out slowly. The pain is often relieved by bladder emptying.

Although the pain is most prominent around the bladder and pelvic region, it is often associated with unexplained widespread body pain. Nearly 50 percent of women and 75 percent of men with UCPPS report chronic pain outside of the pelvic region.[7] Patients with UCPPS have generalized pain sensitivity and pain sensitivity increases during flare-ups of the bladder symptoms. Widespread pain was associated with greater severity of nonpelvic symptoms and poorer psychosocial health but not with worse pelvic pain or bladder symptoms.[8] UCPPS is also associated with increased rates of depression, anxiety, catastrophizing, and perceived stress.[9]

There are changes in brain structure and function suggestive of central sensitization in patients with UCPPS. Unique brain white matter structural changes have correlated with urine proteins that are markers of tissue remodeling.[10] Analogous to the gut-brain axis of IBS, this suggests that the bladder-brain axis promotes the chronic pain in UCPPS.

Susan's multiple diagnoses of IBS, UCPPS, and fibromyalgia are not at all unusual. Somewhere between 30 and 60 percent of fibromyalgia patients will be diagnosed with either IBS, chronic pelvic/bladder pain, or both.[11] Fifty percent of UCPPS patients have fibromyalgia, IBS, or chronic oral/facial pain.[12] The term "functional syndrome" has been used to lump together these

multiple chronic pain conditions with no obvious organic pathology. Some experts have suggested the label of central sensitivity
disorder, the unifying feature being central, rather than peripher-
ally driven, pain.[13]

Each of these disorders was initially categorized by its primary
symptom, according to the usual organic disease model. A fibromyalgia diagnosis is based on musculoskeletal pain, IBS on bowel
pain and change in bowel habits, and chronic pelvic/bladder pain
on urinary frequency/urgency with bladder and pelvic pain. All
subspecialists have focused on their own area of interest and expertise in understanding and treating these seemingly unrelated
pain problems. Rheumatologists are the experts for fibromyalgia,
gastroenterologists for irritable bowel syndrome, and urologists for
chronic pelvic and bladder pain.

In the past, such a specialized, organ-focused approach contributed to ineffective therapy, such as antibiotics for IBS, bladder
or pelvic injections or instillation of various chemicals for chronic
pelvic/bladder pain, or jaw surgery for temporomandibular joint
pain syndrome. Fortunately, most specialists now recognize that
the chronic pain in these conditions is not related to structural
damage and will not respond to organ-based therapy.

Rather than splitting up these chronic pain conditions, we need
to appreciate their common nature. The gastroenterologist, urologist, and I each participated in Susan's ongoing care. I added amitriptyline to her medications. A low dose at bedtime helped her
pain, and when the dose was raised to 50 mg at night, her diarrhea
improved. Susan had avoided intercourse, and this had put added
strain on her marriage. Couples counseling, including advice on
sexual techniques that would decrease the vulvar irritation, were
helpful. The urologist worked with a gynecologist to try approaches to decrease the pelvic sensitivity. Susan found that acupuncture lessened the pelvic irritability. She began a yoga and
physical fitness program. Although she still has exacerbations of
her pelvic pain and urinary frequency, they are much more man-
ageable.

IMPORTANT POINTS ABOUT CHRONIC BLADDER, BOWEL, AND PELVIC PAIN

- Chronic bowel pain with diarrhea or constipation is usually related to irritable bowel syndrome (IBS).
- Chronic pelvic and bladder pain, associated with urinary frequency, urgency, and pelvic sensitivity, is usually caused by urologic chronic pelvic pain syndrome (UCPPS).
- IBS and UCPPS are diagnosed after infection and systemic or structural disease are ruled out, usually after consultation with a gastroenterologist or urologist.
- These conditions overlap with fibromyalgia and other central sensitivity disorders.
- Patient education and treatment should be interdisciplinary within a biopsychological illness model.
- Medications have been approved for diarrhea-predominant IBS and should be used in consultation with a gastroenterologist.

11

ARTHRITIS AND CHRONIC PAIN

I had my first knee surgery when I was thirty-four. It was to remove torn medial meniscus (cartilage), probably the result of playing basketball daily for twenty years. There had been no single injury and, unlike some of my patients, I never felt a "pop" or severe pain. Gradually, the left knee became more painful, and it started to swell after sports. Those were the days before MRIs or arthroscopy. The orthopedic surgeon made a small incision and removed the torn medial meniscus. I hobbled around on crutches, wearing a cast for a few weeks, and gradually the knee felt better.

Over the next twenty-five years the knee continued to be troublesome, and I had two more operations, both arthroscopies. I stopped playing basketball when I was forty-five, stopped squash and tennis by the time I was fifty, and decided to switch from running to biking and swimming. Despite these exercise accommodations, the knee was always painful, and about once a year it would get really swollen. I would ask one of my rheumatology partners to remove the fluid and inject corticosteroids. This would always relieve the acute pain and swelling, but within a few months I was back to square one. Knee X-rays showed that the joint had a lot of arthritis.

Since my patients often had similar stories, I was very familiar with the natural history of knee osteoarthritis (OA). It was only a matter of time until I would need a knee replacement, but I was trying to wait it out. During my long rheumatology career, joint replacement had become more and more successful, but at that time replacements still only lasted ten to fifteen years on average. Therefore, I decided to wait as long as possible.

Finally, I went to consult with one of the most respected knee surgeons in Boston, someone to whom I sent many of my patients for surgery. X-rays now revealed bone-on-bone, advanced arthritis. So I had a total knee replacement at age sixty. The rehabilitation was difficult, but three months postoperatively I was having almost no knee pain, the joint range of motion was normal, and I resumed biking and water exercises. Fifteen years have gone by, and the artificial knee is going strong. The opposite knee, which demonstrated almost as much arthritis on X-ray fifteen years ago, has given me minimal problems.

When people describe chronic pain from arthritis, they usually mean osteoarthritis. OA is by far the most prevalent type of arthritis, affecting thirty million Americans.[1] However, there are more than one hundred different types of arthritis, including those that are part of systemic, immune diseases, such as rheumatoid arthritis (RA) or systemic lupus erythematosus (lupus). Following the antiquated biomedical chronic pain classification, OA has been categorized as a structural pain condition and RA as an inflammatory disease.

Between 10 and 20 percent of Americans will develop painful knee or hip osteoarthritis. Currently almost one million knees and five hundred thousand hips are replaced yearly in the United States.[2] It is estimated that by 2030 three million knee replacements will be done yearly in the United States.[3]

During the past fifty years, osteoarthritis has been considered a disease of wear and tear. This makes perfect sense, since OA slowly advances with age and is more common after repeated joint trauma, resulting in the cartilage, a shock absorber between our joint bones, gradually narrowing. Once the cartilage cushioning wears away, the bones rub against each other, becoming deformed and enlarged. This leads to a grinding noise, called "crepitus," and results in joint pain and decreased joint motion.

I fit the osteoarthritis profile perfectly. I had played a lot of sports that could place physical stress on the knee. We know that basketball players get early osteoarthritis in their knees, and soccer players get it in their ankles. Having the cartilage removed surgically, especially at a young age as I did, also is a risk factor for early knee OA. As we age, the impact of weight bearing will eventually take its toll on all of us, as it did on my knee.

OA advances from the lifelong physical load on our joints. Normal aging is the reason that most of us will have some OA in our knees and hips by age seventy, even if it doesn't bother us much. The increase in obesity in the population has been a prominent factor in the acceleration of rates of knee and hip osteoarthritis.[4] Overweight and obese individuals will require a total knee or hip replacement at a much younger age than normal-weight subjects will.[5] The age for joint replacement correlates with one's level of body mass index (BMI). BMI is derived from each person's weight and height, calculated by weight divided by the square of the height, expressed in kilograms/meter squared (kg/m^2). A BMI of 25–30 is considered overweight, 30–35, moderately obese, and 45–50, morbidly obese. Modestly overweight people are having joint replacement on average seven years earlier than they might otherwise, and severely obese subjects are having joint replacements eleven years earlier than nonoverweight individuals.[6] Fortunately, that was not a factor in my progressive knee arthritis.

In addition to modifiable risk factors for osteoarthritis, like obesity and joint trauma, there are genetic influences for OA. There are rare hereditary forms of OA that begin as early as adolescence, with multiple joints becoming damaged early in adulthood. In most patients, as with each chronic pain condition, hereditary factors are thought to explain 40 to 50 percent of the risk for OA.

Rheumatoid arthritis is the most common inflammatory/immune arthritis. In RA, immune mechanisms, partly genetically determined, incite inflammatory mediators, which result in pain, swelling, and, if unchecked, rapid joint destruction. Since the immune activation can involve every organ in the body, fever, weight loss, and lung, nerve, or even heart inflammation may occur. Normal joint wear and tear is not the main cause of joint damage in RA, and weight-bearing joints are not the most commonly affected. Symmetrical inflammation of the small joints of the hands and feet is classic for RA. Immune activation causing systemic inflammation is characteristic of other rheumatic diseases such as systemic lupus erythematosus, scleroderma, and seronegative spondyloarthropathies. Each of these conditions is usually diagnosed and treated by rheumatologists.

The treatment of RA has always been to block inflammation. When I started out in rheumatology a half century ago, we had few drugs to do that and would often resort to very large doses of aspirin, up to sixteen per day. At these doses, aspirin has a chemical anti-inflammatory effect, whereas you get an analgesic effect from taking just a few aspirin. Corticosteroids, including cortisone, steroids, and prednisone, have a much more powerful anti-inflammatory effect. In 1950 scientists from the Mayo Clinic won the Nobel Prize in Medicine for isolating cortisone and demonstrating its miraculous effect on patients with RA. Unfortunately, severe adverse side effects, including weight gain, swelling, osteoporosis, and cardiac disease, became apparent and precluded taking steroids in high doses for prolonged periods of time. Most importantly, these anti-inflammatory drugs never altered the joint damage to any substantial degree.

Over the years the immune mediators that trigger RA inflammation have been characterized, and drugs have been developed to target and destroy them. Most of the initial immune modulators block a potent stimulator called tumor necrosis factor (TNF). TNF inhibitors, such as Humira and Enbrel, were the first of these immune modulators, but there are now many different classes of chemicals that block various autoimmune targets. These medications are called disease-modifying drugs since that is exactly what they do. In contrast to my early rheumatology career, nowadays I generally can halt the structural joint damage of RA or related immune-systemic diseases with these medicines.

Inflammatory and immune mechanisms are also involved in OA joint damage. However, such immune and inflammatory mediators have not been well characterized, and they may not play a major role in OA joint destruction. Unlike in RA, there are currently no disease-modifying drugs in OA. Treatment has been designed to relieve pain and improve function. For most of the past twenty-five years I have been taking nonsteroidal anti-inflammatory drugs (NSAIDs), as discussed in the next chapter. NSAIDs can also be used topically, and the most popular is diclofenac gel. I got good relief from the knee joint drainage and corticosteroid injections when my knee swelled, but the improvement would only last a few months. An orthopedic surgeon injected my left knee with hyaluronate a few years before my joint replacement. Hyaluronate contains the same substance that lubricates our joints and has been used with limited success in some patients with knee osteoarthritis, but most rheumatology guidelines do not recommend its use.[7] The hyaluronate injection did not help me. Platelet-rich plasma injections have also been popular, but there are no adequate studies to demonstrate that they significantly help pain or limit joint damage.[8]

Millions of people have used supplements to treat their arthritis. The most popular are glucosamine and chondroitin sulfate, two chemicals present in human cartilage. Whether these supplements actually decrease joint pain or lessen OA joint damage has been very controversial. Most studies in the United States have not been positive. European studies have been more favorable, and these differences may relate to the fact that glucosamine and chondroitin sulfate are prescription drugs and regulated in Europe but not in the United States. In one European study, combined glucosamine and chondroitin sulfate were as effective as 200 mg of Celebrex (celecoxib) daily, the NSAID that I have been taking for the past ten years.[9]

One new promising treatment to reduce pain in osteoarthritis is medication that blocks nerve growth factor (NGF). NGF is one of a family of chemicals called "neurotrophins" that are important in peripheral sensory and brain nerve transmission. NGF is produced in excess amounts at sites of tissue injury or damage. A number of antibodies have been developed that block NGF and have been found to be effective in pain reduction in patients with OA. In a recent study, the anti-NGF antibody tanezumab decreased pain and improved function in patients with moderate or severe OA of the knee or hip.[10] These inhibitors of NGF have also shown promise in the treatment of chronic low back pain.

We now realize that the chronic pain in osteoarthritis cannot be explained simply on the basis of structural joint changes. For example, there is poor correlation of the degree of joint damage, seen on X-ray, with pain. Some patients with far advanced knee OA radiologically have little pain, whereas others with minimal evidence of OA on X-ray complain of severe pain. As with every chronic pain condition, central sensitization accounts for much of the variability in pain in OA. Increased generalized pain sensitivity was found in OA patients who had high pain levels yet little radiologic joint damage, whereas those patients with low pain despite advanced X-ray changes had low pain sensitivity.[11] Patients with knee OA have low pain thresholds in many body areas, not just in the bad knee.[12] Differences in gray matter volume, especially in the thalamus, were found in patients with hip OA.[13] One year after hip replacement and pain reduction, the gray matter changes normalized.[14] Similarly, one year after successful knee replacement, preoperative brain imaging evidence that had demonstrated central sensitization completely disappeared.[15] This provides evidence that chronic pain and subsequent neural remapping are strongly related to the OA-damaged knee. Patients with knee OA have twice as much loss of brain gray matter as subjects without chronic pain.[16]

However, chronic pain may persist independent of the severity of joint damage in OA. When patients with knee OA are followed for a number of years, they frequently develop widespread pain, suggestive of fibromyalgia.[17] This has not been associated with a new joint getting OA or severity of the knee OA, suggesting that central sensitization was driving the pain. Depression and sleep disturbances are important factors in OA pain severity. The duration of depression and of sleep disturbances correlates with pain severity over time.[18]

The same central pain factors are important in RA or other forms of systemic arthritis. During my fifty years in rheumatology, I have witnessed amazing progress in the treatment of rheumatoid arthritis. In RA, pinpointing the immune aberrations in the joint and developing drugs to block them led to a complete outcome turnaround. At the start of my career, most patients with RA would end up with severely damaged joints. Now this rarely happens, and joint replacements in RA are not usually needed. Despite these marvelous success stories, at least 25 percent of RA patients have persistent chronic pain. Depression, sleep disorders, and widespread pain sensitivity at nonjoint sites correlate with increased pain and decreased response to medications in patients with RA.[19] Between 20 and 30 percent of RA patients have coexisting fibromyalgia.[20] Neuroimaging in patients with RA reveals changes in regional brain connectivity similar to those in fibromyalgia. Those RA patients with fibromyalgia symptoms score higher on disease activity instruments, which always include questions about pain and fatigue.[21] This leads to the erroneous conclusion that their RA is more active, which is accompanied by a needless increase in immune-targeting medication.

Even when the damaged joint in OA or RA is removed with a surgically successful joint replacement, many patients continue to have chronic, unrelenting pain.[22] That is related to central sensitization. We now recommend that orthopedic surgeons ask their patients about widespread pain, mood, and sleep disturbances prior to surgery. Giving a fibromyalgia questionnaire to patients about to undergo a joint replacement has been used to predict those patients at risk for chronic pain postoperatively. Those patients with more fibromyalgia symptoms had a significantly poorer outcome with greater pain than those with none or few of those symptoms.[23] Fibromyalgia symptoms preoperatively were also associated with greater postoperative opioid use. Central pain must always be kept in mind for optimal medical or surgical outcome.

IMPORTANT POINTS ABOUT CHRONIC PAIN AND ARTHRITIS

- Osteoarthritis is primarily caused by structural joint wear and tear and increases with age, joint trauma, and obesity. Reducing joint load is helpful, but many patients will eventually need a joint replacement.
- Rheumatoid arthritis is caused by immune factors producing joint inflammation. Medicines that target and knock out these abnormalities have been very effective in halting the progression of joint damage.
- Central sensitization is an important factor in arthritis pain and may account for the reason many patients have persistent chronic pain despite optimal medical or surgical management.
- Management of arthritis pain should include an evaluation and treatment for mood and sleep disturbances within a biopsychological illness model.

12

PHARMACOLOGIC THERAPY

Many forms of chronic pain can be treated through the same methods, including similar medications. Classes of medications used to treat chronic pain include nonopioid analgesics, anti-inflammatory drugs, anticonvulsants, antidepressants, topical agents, adjunctive therapies (such as botulinum toxin), and various injections. Opioids and cannabis will be discussed in the next chapter.

Analgesics are pain relievers with no anti-inflammatory effect and are mostly available as over-the-counter (OTC) medications. The only commonly used nonopioid analgesic is Tylenol (acetaminophen). It does not require a prescription and is usually marketed as a 325 mg tablet, with a maximum dose of 4 g per day. Its exact mechanism of action as a pain reliever is not well understood. It has weak analgesic effects, and long-term use of more than 4 g per day is dangerous because of potential liver damage. In the past acetaminophen was often recommended as the first choice for the treatment of chronic pain from a variety of conditions, including osteoarthritis and low back pain, but because of its minimal pain-relieving impact and its potential toxicity, it is no longer commonly used to treat chronic pain. It is the best option for individuals who are allergic to aspirin or other anti-inflammatory medications or for use in lowering fevers.

Nonsteroidal anti-inflammatory drugs (NSAIDs) are the most commonly prescribed pain relievers and many are available without a prescription. Aspirin, generic acetylsalicylic acid (ASA), originally harvested from willow tree leaves, has been used to treat fever and inflammation for more than two thousand years. In 1899 the Bayer pharmaceutical company named ASA "aspirin," and it quickly became the most common medicine prescribed throughout the world.[1] It interferes with platelet function more than any other NSAID, which makes it more likely to cause bleeding. This effect on platelets led to the use of very small amounts of ASA to help prevent heart attacks. ASA and all NSAIDs have an analgesic effect at low doses but at higher doses also have an anti-inflammatory effect. For example, one or two aspirin every four to six hours is recommended for pain reduction, whereas its anti-inflammatory effect requires twelve to fourteen per day. As discussed in the previous chapter, fifty years ago such high doses of aspirin were the mainstay for treating inflammatory forms of arthritis, such as rheumatoid arthritis. However, adverse side effects such as ringing in the ears, gastrointestinal distress, and bleeding were common.

There are many OTC and prescription NSAIDs. Motrin (ibuprofen) and Naprosyn (naproxen) are inexpensive and available OTC. NSAIDs have replaced ASA as the most commonly used pain relievers. For headaches and low back pain, NSAIDs are usually best taken as needed and at the lowest dose that achieves an analgesic effect. In conditions such as rheumatoid arthritis, where inflammation drives the pain, NSAIDs are often used in much higher doses and generally given around the clock.

Corticosteroids, either given orally or by injection, are the most potent anti-inflammatory medications. However, they are not analgesics and are never used solely for pain reduction. They should be used only when pain is the result of local or systemic inflammation. Steroid injections were quite helpful to decrease the pain and swelling from my knee osteoarthritis.

Longer-acting NSAIDs, including diclofenac, sulindac, and nabumetone, are more potent and require less frequent dosing than ibuprofen and naproxen do. However, these require a prescription and will be expensive unless covered by medical insurance plans. There is no good evidence that one NSAID is a more effective pain reliever than another.

All NSAIDs have similar adverse side effects, the most serious being gastrointestinal bleeding and cardiovascular or renal toxicity. Therefore, NSAIDs should be used with caution and with frequent monitoring in elderly patients or those with preexisting cardiac or renal disease.[2] Celebrex (celecoxib) is a selective cyclooxygenase 2 (COX-2) NSAID that has less gastrointestinal toxicity than the nonselective NSAIDs. I have taken celecoxib daily for a number of years in order to decrease pain from my OA. A number of other COX-2 inhibitors were available years ago but were taken off the market because of increased cardiovascular risk. All NSAIDs have a slight increased risk of cardiovascular complications, with naproxen having possibly the least risk.

Many drugs developed to treat neurologic or psychiatric conditions have pain-relieving properties. Anticonvulsants, initially used for the treatment of seizure disorders, have a significant analgesic effect particularly for neuropathic pain, such as diabetic neuropathy. Gabapentin and pregabalin exert their analgesic effect by binding to calcium channels at the alpha 2-delta subunit, thereby inhibiting the release of certain neurotransmitters. They have both been found to relieve pain in fibromyalgia and are the most commonly prescribed drugs for patients with neuropathic pain.[3] Lyrica (pregabalin) is one of just three drugs approved for the treatment of fibromyalgia by the FDA. Anticonvulsants have also been used to treat headaches, low back pain, and chronic bladder and pelvic pain. Their most common adverse side effects include sedation, dizziness, swelling, and weight gain. I often prescribe these medications to be taken at nighttime, to avoid daytime sedation and improve sleep.

A number of antidepressants also have pain-relieving properties. Their analgesic effects are independent of their antidepressant effects. Amitriptyline and other so-called tricyclic antidepressants have been used for the treatment of neuropathic pain and low back pain and have been extensively studied in the treatment of fibromyalgia. The average doses used to treat pain have been much lower than the doses used to treat depression. In fibromyalgia, Elavil (amitriptyline) has usually been used at very low doses, 10 to 30 mg, at bedtime. The first RCT we did in Boston was to compare 25 mg of amitriptyline, given at bedtime, to anti-inflammatory doses of ibuprofen.[4] The amitriptyline improved pain and overall well-being better than the ibuprofen and much better than placebo. Flexeril (cyclobenzaprine), a similar medication, is marketed as a muscle relaxant but works like amitriptyline. Common side effects of these tricyclic compounds include sedation, dry mouth, and constipation. These side effects, as well as mental confusion, are especially prominent in elderly patients. If the dose is kept low, such as 10 to 30 mg of Elavil at bedtime, these side effects are usually not worrisome.

The most commonly prescribed antidepressants are serotonin-reuptake inhibitors (SSRIs), such as Prozac (fluoxetine) and Zoloft (sertraline). These medications have minimal analgesic effect on their own, but when we combined low doses of fluoxetine in the morning with low doses of amitriptyline at bedtime, patients with fibromyalgia had significant pain relief.[5] A different class of antidepressants, serotonin norepinephrine reuptake inhibitors (SNRIs), do have more potent pain-relieving impact. Two of them, Cymbalta (duloxetine) and Savella (milnacipran) have been approved for the treatment of fibromyalgia, and Cymbalta is also approved for the treatment of osteoarthritis. These medications have also been used in the treatment of neuropathic pain.

Tramadol is a pain-reliever classified as a weak opioid, but most of its pain-relieving effect is related to serotonin inhibition. It has less addiction potential than strong opioids but still is potentially capable of causing drug dependence. It has been used alone and in combination with acetaminophen and showed modest pain reduction in fibromyalgia. However, the use of tramadol in patients with OA was associated with increased mortality compared to those treated only with NSAIDs.[6]

Topical medications have the advantage of less systemic side effects and can be particularly helpful when the pain is confined to a single anatomic site. The most common include capsaicin and topical lidocaine, which is an anesthetic, like most of the topical pain relievers advertised on television. IcyHot, the pain reliever that basketball great Shaquille O'Neal promotes, is lidocaine and comes in a patch or spray. Capsaicin is derived from chili peppers and works on peripheral nerve endings. It is available as a cream and a patch and has shown promise as an injectable drug in OA. Almost every pain medication can be compounded into a topical agent; however, the standardization of these products is often poor.

Topical NSAIDs can be effective in localized joint or muscle pain. Topical diclofenac was as effective as oral diclofenac with less adverse side effects in patients with pain related to knee OA.[7] Topical gabapentin and high doses of topical capsaicin have been used to treat neuropathic pain. Topical agents that have been touted to treat pain with minimal evidence for their efficacy include creams containing glucosamine and chondroitin, menthol, herbal therapies, and salvia extract.

There is a wide array of injectable medications used for the treatment of chronic pain. Botulinum toxin (BTX or Botox) interferes with the release of pain neurotransmitters and can downregulate peripheral and central pain sensitization. As an injectable drug, it reduces neuropathic pain and pain associated with migraine. It has been used for the prevention of chronic migraine where it is thought to inhibit the release of calcitonin gene-related peptide (CGRP) from peripheral neurons. Botox is also used in cosmetic procedures to minimize the appearance and development of new wrinkles.

Epidural steroid injections are commonly used for the treatment of back pain, with or without concurrent sciatica, and can be quite effective in carefully selected patients. The same is true of injections of local anesthetic agents in peripheral nerves or around vertebral nerves, termed "facet joint nerve blocks."

Unfortunately, most currently available analgesics are not very effective in relieving chronic pain. This has led to the practice of combining different classes of these medications. For example,

NSAIDs may be used along with an anticonvulsant in the treatment of a peripheral neuropathy. In fibromyalgia, rather than pushing a single medication to the maximum tolerated dose, I often recommend combining two medications. A common regimen might include a serotonin/norepinephrine reuptake inhibitor in the morning and an anticonvulsant in the evening. This takes advantage of each drug's distinctive analgesic action and also the fact that their side effect profiles are different. Pharmaceutical companies have marketed a number of drugs that combine different analgesic effects in a single tablet, such as a drug containing both acetaminophen and ibuprofen. However, such combinations eliminate the ability to gauge the potency or toxicity of the two distinct chemical compounds.

There is a desperate need for new, more effective and better targeted pain relievers. Specificity is dependent on a better understanding of disease mechanisms. Migraine medications have evolved through researchers' greater appreciation of the neural mechanisms involved in initiating and perpetuating migraine. In the previous chapter, I discussed the anti-NGF medications that look very promising for the treatment of OA and low back pain. These are novel analgesics, targeting a newly described pain-promoting factor. The FDA has been very cautious about its appoval of anti-NGF drugs because of concern about rare but very real bone damage. Opioids that target delta and kappa receptors rather than mu receptors are also being tested. The hope is that they may be safer and less addicting.

The effectiveness of any pain reliever may differ depending on the predominant mechanism of chronic pain. Anticonvulsants are more effective for neuropathic pain than for musculoskeletal pain. However, since central sensitization plays an important role in all chronic pain, it often is impossible to classify the dynamics behind any individual's chronic pain. Most often trial and error will be required to find a medication or a combination of medications with the best pain relief and the least adverse side effects. Pain medications work best when given as part of multidisciplinary management, to include exercise and behavioral modification.

Relying solely on killing the pain resulted too often in killing the patients, and it led to our opioid crisis, to be discussed next.

IMPORTANT POINTS ABOUT PAIN MEDICATIONS

- Analgesics, like acetaminophen, are weak pain relievers.
- Anti-inflammatory medications, including aspirin and NSAIDs, are the most commonly prescribed pain medications.
- Topical NSAIDs, anesthetics, and capsaicin have no significant internal absorption and may be preferable when the pain is limited to small regions.
- Injections of steroids or anesthetic agents in and around joints, nerves, and soft tissue may be helpful in carefully selected patients.
- Pain relievers with different mechanisms of action, when combined, can complement each other.
- Certain chronic pain conditions may respond better to certain classes of pain relievers.

13

THE OPIOID CRISIS; CANNABIS

OPIOIDS

Opioids are a group of substances that exert their powerful analgesic effect by binding to opioid receptors found in the brain,
spinal cord, and gut. Originally derived from a resin in the opium
poppy, hence the term *opioids*, they were hailed as the "plant of
joy" in the fourth century BCE and used by Hippocrates to treat
pain.[1] From the fifteenth century to the nineteenth century, a
number of opium compounds were widely used and available le-
gally and illegally.[2] At the turn of the nineteenth century, morphine was isolated from the opium plant and hailed as a wonder
drug with no addiction potential. Codeine was then extracted from
opium, and shortly thereafter scientists began making synthetic
opioids, including Demerol and heroin.[3]

Our bodies produce endogenous opioids—including endorphins, which are activated in the "runner's high." Opioids bind to
one of three receptors in the brain, mu, kappa, or delta, and the
potency as well as the toxicity of synthetic opioids is dependent on
this binding. Opioids' pain-relieving effect is primarily related to
its mu receptor binding. This binding also results in opioids' eu-
phoric effects, although a number of brain receptors are involved
in their many psychoactive properties. As new opioids were manu-

factured, their potency dramatically increased. Morphine is the standard, with a relative potency of 1, whereas the potency of other synthetically manufactured opioids like fentanyl is 100 and Carfentanil, a synthetic derivative of fentanyl, is 1000.[4] Unfortunately, as the potency has increased, so, too, have each opioid's addictive properties. Fentanyl comes in a patch (Duragesic) as well as in a lollipop or lozenge. These formulations were meant for cancer patients with severe pain but have found their way to the street drug market. There are now many illicitly manufactured analogues of fentanyl, all hundreds of times more potent that heroin.

A 2016 *Time* magazine article, "Heroin Is Being Laced with a Terrifying New Substance," publicized the surge of deaths from Carfentanil usually of drug users who thought they were taking heroin.[5] In one week in Hamilton County, Ohio, there were one hundred deaths from Carfentanil that was mixed in with heroin unbeknown to the users. Carfentanil is easier to make and less expensive to buy than heroin is. It is five thousand times as potent as heroin, and just a few granules the size of table salt can be fatal.

Opioids are effective pain relievers and the drug of choice for severe, acute pain and for cancer patients with significant pain. Their sedative and psychoactive effects have made them important as anesthetic agents but also highly addictive, so they usually are called narcotics. The term *narcotic* is derived from words suggesting sleep and numbness. Opioids' psychoactive effect is the mechanism leading to opioid-induced tolerance and dependence as well as to addiction. It also drives the reward sensation induced by opioids, an important part of the craving for opioids. Tolerance, the body's normal adaptation to a drug's influence, eventually causes the body to require a higher dose to get the same pain-relieving result. Dependence is defined by the occurrence of withdrawal symptoms when the opioid is abruptly discontinued or the dose decreased. Neither drug tolerance nor dependence necessarily results in addiction.[6] The vast majority of people who take prescription opioids do not become addicted. However, if the opioid is continued long-term, increasingly higher doses will be needed for the same pain reduction. This can also result in opioid-induced hyperalgesia, a form of generalized pain hypersensitivity with similar neurobiological changes as noted in conditions such as fibromyalgia.

Opioid addiction is a complex state of physical signs and compulsive psychological behavior, resulting in personal and societal harm and drug abuse.[7] Addiction is usually associated with illicit drug use as a diversion. There are genetic and environmental risk factors for addiction that are similar to those discussed for chronic pain. Structural and functional brain alterations, particularly involving emotional circuitry, are present in individuals with drug addiction. Opioid tolerance, dependence, and addiction are central to the opioid crisis in the United States.

Until the 1980s, opioids were prescribed primarily for the treatment of acute pain. This changed dramatically when pharmaceutical companies began aggressively promoting opioids for the treatment of chronic, noncancer-related pain. Opioid prescriptions increased from 71 million per year in 1991 to 290 million in 2016.[8] Opioid analgesics became the most commonly prescribed class of medications in the United States, and Americans became the largest per-capita consumer of opioids in the world. This led to the addiction of more than 2.5 million Americans, with 70,000 drug overdose deaths yearly.[9] The majority of these deaths are related to illicit drug use, but a significant proportion of drug abusers' first exposure to opioids was from a physician-prescribed drug. One hundred Americans die daily from opioid overdose, and 50 percent of those are linked to a prescribed opioid.[10]

A number of pharmaceutical companies contributed to the opioid crisis, but Purdue Pharma's promotion and marketing of Oxy-Contin has been the most blatant. From 1995 to 2010 Purdue conducted many national, all-expenses-paid pain-management conferences for more than five thousand physicians, each trained to join Purdue's speaker bureau, where they were provided with educational materials and slides developed by Purdue.[11] Purdue targeted physicians who were the largest opioid prescribers and paid them handsomely to be the company's spokespersons. Purdue also greatly increased their sales representatives and provided all physicians with free seven- to thirty-day prescriptions to start their patients on OxyContin. Purdue coached their sales representatives and physicians in the outright lie that the risk of addiction from OxyContin was "less than one percent."[12] Sales of OxyContin grew from $48 million in 1996 to 1.1 billion in 2000.[13]

I have seen firsthand how opioid addiction destroys families. Cindy, the daughter of one of my patients, had been very popular in high school, an honors student, until she began dealing with body image issues and anorexia. After seeing a number of mental health professionals, her anorexia got under control, but she began having severe back and pelvic pain. She was given a prescription for OxyContin by her family physician. Over the next few months, Cindy became dependent on that drug, but her doctor refused to continue the prescription. Desperate, she stole one of her mother's outdated codeine bottles until those ran dry. After a few months she was addicted to heroin. Cindy has been shooting up heroin for the past three years, either living on the street or being secluded at home. During that time Cindy has been in and out of detox at least five times. Her mother, a patient I had been treating for rheumatoid arthritis, was in tears each time I saw her during the ensuing few years. It became much more difficult to control her rheumatoid arthritis. At the mom's last visit, we were talking about our children and she achingly cried out, "I keep telling Cindy how much I love her, knowing each day it might be the last thing I say to her."

In addition to their addiction potential, we now know that opioids are no better for chronic pain relief than nonopioid analgesics. In the largest systematic analysis yet published, opioids were compared to nonopioid pain treatments for more than twenty-six thousand patients with a variety of chronic pain conditions.[14] There was similar improvement in pain and functioning when comparing opioids with nonopioid analgesics, including NSAIDs and tricyclic antidepressants. These results were limited to clinical trials of one to six months. There was even less pain relief when opioids were evaluated in trials lasting six months, possibly related to opioid-induced hyperalgesia. These studies also excluded patients with current or prior substance abuse or an active mental health disorder, situations where chronic opioid use is particularly likely to be problematic.

Current clinical practice guidelines discourage long-term opioid use for headache, low back pain, or fibromyalgia. In fact, in fibromyalgia there is evidence that chronic opioid therapy interferes with benefits from multidimensional therapy and increases harms, including sexual dysfunction, cardiovascular disease, and suicide.[15] Whenever a trial of an opioid is considered for noncancer chronic pain, the potential risks and benefits should be reviewed, and the opioids should be continued only after a well-documented benefit has been achieved. Buprenorphine is considered to be less habit-forming than other long-acting opioids. It is also one of three drugs, along with methadone and naltrexone, that can treat opioid-use disorder. If opioids are prescribed, they should be used short-term and with the expectation of transition to nonopioid chronic pain management. The opioid crisis in the United States has taught us that harms from these drugs outweigh their benefit in the treatment of chronic pain conditions, although they continue to be appropriate in the treatment of acute pain, cancer-related pain, or intractable pain.

CANNABIS

Cannabis, popularly known as marijuana, has been used for medicinal reasons for thousands of years. It is a plant-derived cannabinoid. Cannabinoids are chemicals present in plants but also in humans. Our body's cannabinoids regulate various organ functions and have been implicated in a number of diseases, including migraine and depression. Like opioid receptors, there are cannabinoid receptors throughout the body, and, like opioids, they are important in pain neuropathways. Cannabis and its various components can be derived from plants or made synthetically. Cannabis's psychoactive effects are linked to one cannabinoid, delta-9-

tetrahydrocannabinol (THC). Its analgesic effects are mainly due to cannabidiol (CBD). CBD is usually extracted from hemp, a cannabis plant that also contains tiny amounts of THC. CBD inhibits neurotransmitters and neuropeptides involved in pain processing.[16] CBD also has anti-inflammatory effects.

There are now hundreds of cannabis products available for recreational or medical use. However, there are no consistent formulations nor effective regulation of these compounds. Therefore it is very difficult to know the potency or purity of these substances. Some of the synthetic cannabinoids have been developed to target disease states, including chronic pain. Epidiolex is a CBD extract that has been approved by the FDA for the treatment of epilepsy.[17] Nabiximols, a generic name for cannabis extracts, have been approved in the UK to treat neuropathic pain and other symptoms associated with multiple sclerosis.[18] Nabilone, one of these cannabis extracts, was found to be helpful for sleep but not for pain, in a trial in patients with fibromyalgia and other rheumatic diseases.[19] CBD compounds have also been effective in treating cancer-related pain, most often in combination with opioids. The efficacy of these compounds in noncancer-related pain is less clear. In a systematic analysis of 16 medical studies with 1,750 patients, a number of cannabis-based medications were found to have minimal pain reduction in patients with chronic neuropathic pain, and adverse side effects outweighed any benefit.[20]

The approval and marketing of medical and recreational marijuana in many states has driven consumer demand but has complicated any meaningful consensus regarding its role in chronic pain management. Recently, one of my favorite football players, Rob Gronkowski, was touting CBD oil on television and in the press. He claimed it had knocked out most of the chronic unrelenting pain from his multiple football injuries. This may be true, but he was being paid a tidy sum by the CBD manufacturer. It is likely that topical CBD will be less effective for chronic pain than ingested or inhaled formulations, but its popularity is soaring.

Any beneficial effects from cannabis on chronic pain, poor sleep, and anxiety seem more related to CBD than THC. We need more studies of various cannabis products in all chronic pain conditions, including migraine and low back pain. On September 24, 2019, the Arthritis Foundation, on its website, https://www. arthritis.org, issued the first national guideline for CBD guidance, noting, "We are intrigued by the potential of CBD to help people find pain relief and are on record urging the FDA to expedite the study and regulation of these products. There are no established clinical guidelines to inform usage. Experts recommend starting with a low dose, and if relief is inadequate, increase in small increments weekly. Buy from a reputable company that has each batch tested for purity, potency, and safety by an independent laboratory and provides a certificate of analysis."

There is a general consensus that cannabis is less likely to cause drug tolerance, dependence, and addiction than opioids are. However, cannabis has psychoactive properties, and it is possible that its perceived benefit in pain patients may derive more from its high than from its analgesic properties. This is especially concerning in younger individuals where marijuana has had an adverse effect on cognitive development and has been found to be a predictor of opioid use and abuse.[21] A recent report found that in patients with chronic pain, low daily use of cannabis was more effective for pain reduction and safer than high daily use.[22] Initially there was encouraging evidence that the greater accessibility of cannabis could help stem the opioid crisis, including a study reporting that states that had passed medical marijuana laws saw a 25 percent reduction in deaths from opioids.[23] However, more recent studies came to the opposite conclusion, finding an increase in opioid-related deaths in cannabis users.[24] Although cannabis-related products, particularly CBD, seem promising for the treatment of chronic pain, much more research is needed to turn hype into hope.

**IMPORTANT POINTS ABOUT OPIOIDS AND
CANNABIS FOR CHRONIC PAIN**

• Opioids should not be prescribed for most patients with chronic
  pain because of the risk of addiction and harmful side effects,
  and the evidence shows that they are no more effective than
  nonopioid analgesics.
• Opioids are appropriate for acute pain and treatment of pain in
  patients with cancer. In other situations, they should only be
  used along with multidisciplinary management and with the expectation of transition to nonopioid analgesics.
• Cannabis products, particularly CBD, have potential as relative-
  ly safe and effective pain medication, but more long-term studies are needed.

14

EXERCISE

I am addicted to exercise. At least there are a lot of worse things to be addicted to. During each of my injuries, illnesses, and operations, forced inactivity got me down. As quickly as possible, I needed to resume my daily exercise in order to recover physically and emotionally. My brain is accustomed to those added endorphins that accompany my workouts.

There is overwhelming evidence that exercise is beneficial for the treatment of chronic pain. The most extensively studied form of exercise is cardiovascular fitness training. However, all forms of aerobic and resistance or stretching exercises, as well as tai chi and yoga, result in pain reduction. The greater the exercise intensity and duration, the more pain relief is achieved.[1]

Exercise activates multiple endogenous systems involved in pain transmission, with the resultant release of opioids, serotonin, cannabinoids, noradrenaline, and anti-inflammatory cytokines.[2] Following exercise, pain tolerance for pressure or heat increases.[3] In patients with chronic pain, including fibromyalgia, moderate-intensity cycling improved pain ratings, and there was improvement in centrally mediated pain control, based on functional imaging changes in the insula and in brain connectivity.[4] Aerobic exercise has a strong impact on the brain's opioid receptors, considered to be a dominant mechanism of the "runner's high."[5]

Exercise not only decreases pain but also improves cognitive and psychological health. Chronic pain interferes with cognitive ability and is a risk factor for dementia. In a large population-based study, chronic pain was associated with depression, memory decline, and dementia in subjects ages sixty-seven to seventy-eight.[6] Increased aerobic fitness is associated with greater white- and gray-matter brain volume and better communication between brain regions important in pain, cognition, mood, and sleep.[7] Aerobic exercise increases overall brain volume and can attenuate the normal loss of hippocampal brain volume that occurs with aging.[8] One study followed 3,247 adults, ages eighteen to thirty, over twenty-five years.[9] Those who did not engage in regular moderate physical activity had worse executive function and lower brain-processing speed in midlife. Physical activity also leads to social interactions, which promotes cognitive engagement.

Aerobic exercise decreases pain and improves function and quality of life in patients with fibromyalgia.[10] In a study from Spain, more than four hundred women with fibromyalgia were closely evaluated after they did light or moderate aerobic exercise for thirty minutes a few times per week instead of being sedentary.[11] This modest exercise decreased their pain and improved their physical and social function. There was also significant improvement in sleep and fatigue. The fibromyalgia patients who achieved the highest level of physical fitness had the most improvement in pain reduction and quality of life. Aerobic exercise decreased pain and improved both physical and psychological function and well-being in patients with chronic low back pain as well as in patients with chronic pelvic pain.[12] Although intense exercise may, in some people, precipitate a migraine attack, regular exercise decreases the frequency of attacks.[13]

Any form of movement as opposed to being sedentary should be encouraged. You might start simply by taking stairs instead of an elevator or walking a few blocks instead of driving. Gradually the exercise should be aerobic, defined as any physical exercise of low to moderate intensity over a sufficient period of time that utilizes oxygen substantially more than at rest. Anaerobic exercise, such as intense strength-training and sprinting, increases oxygen debt, particularly involving muscle contractions. Therefore, anaerobic exercise is not usually recommended for treating chronic pain. Many forms of exercise involve both aerobic and anaerobic metabolism. The initial focus for treating chronic pain should be on gradual, incremental aerobic activity. The most common aerobic exercises are walking, jogging, cycling, and swimming. Water or land aerobic classes, dancing, rowing, and sports such as tennis are popular aerobic activities. Resistance training and flexibility exercises have shown efficacy in every chronic pain disorder. Resistance training does not mean that you have to lift a lot of weights; rather, it can employ many modalities and can be done in the water as well as on land.

Pilates, originally developed by Joseph Pilates in the 1940s, focuses on the core muscles of the abdomen, low back, and hips to increase strength, balance, and coordination. They may be done on a mat or with a specialized apparatus known as a reformer. They have been particularly effective in the treatment of chronic low back pain.[14]

The specific aerobic exercise should be chosen based on one's interest, level of fitness, and age. It should be started slowly but gradually increased to two or three times weekly, and it needs to be continued for at least twelve weeks for any meaningful pain improvement. A goal should be thirty to sixty minutes of low- to moderate-intensity exercise at 60 to 70 percent of maximum heart rate. Maximum heart rate in beats per minute is estimated at 220 beats minus your age. So, if you are forty, your maximum heart rate would be 180, and ideally you would keep your heart rate between 100 and 125 beats per minute for aerobic fitness training. The exercise can be broken up into shorter sessions, but at least thirty minutes per session is ideal.

Depending on current activity and fitness levels and age, it is often helpful to see a physical therapist prior to beginning an exercise program. This is especially important in individuals with chronic pain related to an injury or with more localized, chronic neck or back pain. A physical therapist is trained to provide you with an exercise program tailored to your current physical status and can best advise you on how to work with any limitations. Physical therapists use a variety of techniques to increase mobility with guided stretching and target areas in need of strengthening.

I have often recommended that my patients begin water-based exercises, such as swimming, water aerobics, and water-resistance training. Simply walking up and down the lane in water can be a good way to start. Personally, I have become very enamored with water aerobics, which I do at least twice weekly. Most water aerobics classes integrate cardiovascular fitness training with stretching and resistance exercises. Exercising in the water tends to be less stressful on our joints and especially suitable for overweight or older individuals and people with osteoarthritis. In a long-term, prospective study on 2,637 individuals, swimming was found to be protective against knee pain and knee OA.[15]

There has been a long-running debate about whether running leads to more knee and hip pain and degenerative arthritis. I switched from running to swimming when I was fifty for just that reason. Most long-range studies have not found an increase in knee or hip OA in runners compared to nonrunners.[16] Self-selected bias may be involved in these studies since people who continue to run may have different body types than those who find running more painful, as I did. Nevertheless, even in people with some knee pain and early arthritis, running at lower intensity, and less often, is recommended.[17]

A sedentary lifestyle predisposes to chronic pain, irrespective of body mass. High body mass index (BMI) and obesity are major risk factors for chronic pain. Obese adults have twice the rate of chronic pain and more severe pain than normal weight adults.[18] Obesity, defined as a BMI of over 30, was the greatest risk factor for chronic pain in a study of 1,500 adults ages sixty-two to eighty-six.[19] Young adults on a weight gain trajectory toward obesity were much more likely to develop chronic pain than those with a high-normal or normal expected weight gain.[20]

It makes perfect sense that since obesity increases the load on our bodies, it would increase the risk of pain and structural damage in weight-bearing joints, such as the knee, hip, or back. The prevalence of low back pain increases as the BMI rises. Less than 3 percent of adults with a normal BMI have chronic low back pain compared to 12 percent who are obese.[21] Pain doesn't just increase in weight-bearing joints with obesity, but we know that obesity increases pain severity in fibromyalgia, chronic headaches, and irritable bowel syndrome.[22] This may relate to the role of obesity in increasing generalized pain sensitivity or to other factors such as increased sleep and mood disturbances. Between 25 and 60 percent of women with fibromyalgia are obese. In a study of 123 obese fibromyalgia patients, those who lost at least 10 percent of their body weight showed greater improvement in pain and other symptoms.[23]

Aerobic exercise, along with a balanced diet, is the cornerstone for weight reduction. However, significant weight loss without caloric restriction is unlikely unless the aerobic activity is very intense.[24] Regular and moderate aerobic activity may promote modest weight loss of about 2 kg over a few months. A combination of aerobic and resistance exercise with weight loss is the best approach to treating anyone with chronic pain, particularly older individuals.[25]

I first met Andrew when he was thirty-eight; he came to see me because of incapacitating chronic knee and hip pain. Andrew was morbidly obese and could barely move, even when supported by his walker. There was a family history of obesity, and Andrew was fully aware of the fact that his weight had destroyed his joints. X-rays revealed far advanced OA in both knees and both hips.

Andrew had been told that he needed these joints to be replaced, but no orthopedic surgeon was willing to do that until he lost a huge amount of weight. He had been going to Weight Watchers and following a strict diet but had only lost 30 pounds during the previous two years. When I met Andrew, he weighed 360 pounds. There was almost no range of motion in either hip, and he could not bend his knees more than thirty degrees.

Andrew had been to our weight loss clinic and advised to have gastric bypass surgery. He had heard a bunch of "horror stories about the bypass" and was afraid of its complications. I tried to assuage his fears, but he was not willing to consider the surgery.

During the next year Andrew worked diligently on further weight loss and did water exercises for two hours every other day. When I saw him a year later, he had lost another fifty pounds, but there was no letup in the pain. We discussed his plight in great detail. Andrew was caught in a catch-22. He was unable to increase his activity levels or exercise because of his arthritis but was told he could not have the joint replacement surgery because of the obesity.

Some orthopedic specialists are willing to operate even in patients with advanced knee or hip OA who have a BMI greater than 40 kg/m^2, and these patients' complication rate of 4 percent is only slightly higher than in nonobese patients.[26] However, studies have shown that withholding joint replacements from the morbidly obese patient does not incentivize significant weight loss.[27] Among the 20 percent of morbidly obese patients who do undergo total joint replacements, the majority have remained morbidly obese.[28] Andrew and I went over the findings from studies demonstrating that morbidly obese patients who have bypass or other bariatric surgery have much better long-term results from joint replacements.[29] He had a successful gastric bypass and lost another sixty pounds. One year later he had both hips replaced and plans to have the knees replaced in the next few years.

You should consider exercise as a prescription to treat chronic pain, the prescription with the least likelihood of adverse side effects. You would not stop a medicine that is working, and the same goes for exercise. Too often my patients begin an exercise program in good faith but don't continue with it. Various forms of exercise complement each other. Your exercise routine should include low-impact cardiovascular fitness training, stretching, and resistance training. My personal lifelong obsession with exercise and physical fitness has evolved and become less driven and healthier. This wasn't purposeful but was the result of my body changing as I aged, had numerous illnesses and injuries, and eventually needed a knee replacement and a back fusion. I am content with taking a long walk with my dog rather than competing with thirtysomethings in a cycling class. Each morning, I do simple yoga poses—really just stretching out on a mat. For the past twenty years, most of the aerobic and strengthening exercise that I do has been in the water. Each of us should find the exercise routine that works best for us, be willing to mix it up and make adjustments to it, and, most importantly, stick with it.

IMPORTANT POINTS ABOUT EXERCISE AND CHRONIC PAIN

- Exercise decreases chronic pain and improves sleep, mood, and cognition.
- Cardiovascular fitness exercise gives the best results, but strength training, flexibility exercises, and Pilates have efficacy in certain pain disorders.
- Physical therapists or rehabilitation specialists can help guide your exercise choice, particularly when there is localized pain or injury.
- Obesity is a major risk factor for chronic pain and inactivity and is best treated with integrated weight-loss programs and low-impact cardiovascular exercise.
- When embarking on an exercise regimen, start gradually, try different forms of exercise, and adjust as needed.

15

COMPLEMENTARY AND ALTERNATIVE MEDICINE, INCLUDING YOGA, TAI CHI, AND ACUPUNCTURE

Complementary medicine is usually defined as any health care that is an adjunct to traditional therapy. Complementary health care for chronic pain includes mainstream techniques such as tai chi, yoga, acupuncture, and massage. There is considerable evidence that each of these can be helpful in the treatment of chronic pain. Herbal and other dietary products, including nutraceuticals, sometimes are considered complementary but are best thought of in the category of alternative medicine. Alternative medicine is generally employed as a substitute to traditional health care. Chiropractic care is also often classified within complementary medicine but may be more alternative, depending on individual practice style.

Complementary health care is used by about 40 percent of the US population each year.[1] Complementary medicine use is twice as high in people with chronic pain than in the general population.[2] The most common forms of complementary or alternative medicine include dietary interventions and herbal or natural products.[3] About fifteen million adults use complementary medicine for the treatment of chronic low back pain.[4] Approximately \$8.5

billion out of pocket is spent on complementary medicine yearly by Americans to manage back pain and \$3.6 billion to manage neck pain.[5]

There are wide variations not just in the United States but throughout the world in the training and regulation of complementary medicine practitioners, as well as in their procedures and products. In many countries, acupuncture can only be performed by physicians. The same holds true for naturopaths. Chiropractors in the United States may focus on musculoskeletal pain, but some may claim to treat cancer and systemic diseases. As discussed in chapter 11, glucosamine and chondroitin sulfate are prescribed medicines in Europe but are over-the-counter supplements in the United States.

The use of tai chi, yoga, and qigong has tripled in the United States during the past ten years. Chronic pain has been the most common reason cited by participants for beginning these exercise programs.[6] Tai chi, yoga, and qigong all employ gentle, flowing body movement with deep breathing and relaxation techniques. They have been shown to improve aerobic fitness, muscle conditioning, and flexibility. Their efficacy in chronic pain conditions may derive from their tamping down central nervous system irritability, as highlighted in the next chapter on mind-body therapy. For example, yoga often lowers blood pressure and decreases the heart rate but primarily when the practice has included meditation.[7]

Tai chi, which began as a martial art, is now practiced throughout the world for its health benefits. It utilizes specified movements and postures with a focus on breathing, calmness, and repetition. Qigong is closely related and considered by some to be a form of tai chi dedicated totally to health and meditation.

Our research group in Boston did one of the initial controlled trials of tai chi in fibromyalgia patients, which was subsequently published in the prestigious *New England Journal of Medicine*.[8] In that study, sixty-six fibromyalgia patients were treated either with a three-month program of supervised tai chi classes or with education and discussion classes. Those who practiced tai chi had significantly less pain, better function, and better overall well-being. Tai chi was also found to be comparable to aerobic exercise for improving the symptoms of fibromyalgia, also effective for treating chronic low back and neck pain, and very cost-effective.[9] Brain neuroimaging has revealed that tai chi leads to decreased central sensitization, very similar to that observed after aerobic exercise.[10]

Yoga includes a spiritual and a mental, as well as a physical, practice. In the Western world we usually consider yoga to be a form of exercise, most often called hatha yoga. Yoga uses postures or poses, called asanas, to improve physical fitness and achieve relaxation and stress reduction. Different schools and styles of yoga have been used in studies on chronic pain, the most frequent an unbranded form of hatha yoga combining a series of postures with meditation and deep breathing. Iyengar yoga, which emphasizes slow postural alignment, can be particularly well suited for patients in chronic pain since it uses props and bolsters to achieve proper positioning without undue strain on the body.

There is moderate evidence that yoga is helpful in patients with chronic low back pain.[11] An eight-week yoga program improved pain, catastrophizing, and function in patients with fibromyalgia.[12] Yoga also improved pain and quality of life in women with chronic pelvic pain.[13] Yoga has been shown to increase heat and pressure pain tolerance, demonstrating its impact on abnormal pain processing.[14]

Acupuncture has been used to treat fibromyalgia, chronic low back and neck pain, CRPS, migraine, and osteoarthritis. In most studies acupuncture has resulted in moderate pain reduction and has been better than sham acupuncture, in which the acupuncture needles are inserted at nontraditional sites.[15] Acupuncture has been studied most extensively in chronic low back pain and fibromyalgia.[16]

Traditional acupuncture involves inserting tiny needles into specific locations. Electroacupuncture uses electrical current instead of plain needle insertion. The classic Chinese teaching is that acupuncture works by redirecting the biologic energy in meridian body channels, balancing yin and yang. There is no scientific evidence for the existence of such energy channels, and many acupuncturists believe that its analgesic effect relates to stimulation of sensory nerve fibers. New research has found that acupuncture's pain reduction is a consequence of central nervous system pain modification. A series of neuroimaging studies found that acupuncture increased the functional connectivity of nerve transmission within pain-controlling regions in the brain.[17]

Various massage therapies have been evaluated in patients with chronic pain. Swedish massage of various lengths of time over eight weeks decreased pain in knee OA, most notably in patients who had received the longest duration of massage, which was six hundred total minutes.[18] Massage has been best evaluated in a number of reports in patients with chronic back or neck pain.[19] The results were generally positive, especially when more sessions were used and when patients also performed self-massage.

Osteopathy originally began as an alternative to traditional medicine and was based on manipulating joints and bones to diagnose and treat diseases. Over the past fifty years it has evolved to become almost indistinguishable from traditional allopathic medicine. Osteopaths, credentialed as DOs rather than MDs, now have similar disease approaches and training to that of traditional medicine, including four years of medical school followed by residency training. Osteopathic physicians are licensed to perform medicine and surgery in every state.

In contrast, chiropractors have persisted in their belief that the musculoskeletal system is the source of many diseases. Chiropractors have usually based their treatments on supposed vertebral joint misalignments, erroneously labeled vertebral subluxations. However, vertebrae and bones don't misalign unless there is major trauma. The training and regulation of chiropractors vary considerably. Most Americans use chiropractors to treat neck or back pain. Whether spinal manipulation works better than other forms of physical therapy remains controversial. There is no evidence that chiropractic treatment is beneficial for any systemic disease.

Most studies of chiropractic vary considerably in the type of manipulation that was done and whether performed by licensed osteopaths, chiropractors, or physical therapists. There is some poor-quality evidence that spinal manipulation or other forms of chiropractic treatment can help chronic low back or neck pain.[20] One of the physical therapists who has worked with a lot of my patients over the years uses spinal manipulation as part of his treatment in some patients. He "cracked my back" a few times along with other, more standard physical therapy when my chronic back pain acted up. I thought the manipulations helped ease my pain. Maybe it was a placebo effect?

Various forms of heat and cold may help acute pain, but there is little evidence that they help chronic pain. There are some studies that demonstrate benefit from hydrotherapy, including in patients with fibromyalgia and chronic low back pain. There is less evidence for any pain-relieving effects from cryotherapy. When my chronic pain flares up, I always find relief from soaking in a hot tub or getting in a whirlpool. Who cares if there is no conclusive evidence? We all know it helps relieve our aches and pains.

The most common form of complementary or alternative medicine is the use of dietary intervention: herbal products and vitamins. Migraine is the one chronic pain condition in which diet and certain additives may precipitate or aggravate pain, as reviewed in chapter 6. There have been claims made about gluten-free, aspartame-free, and vegetarian diets with regard to chronic pain, but there's no conclusive evidence that they help reduce pain severity.[21] Omega-3 supplements, Chinese herbal medicine, and garlic have been advocated for pain reduction, but there are no adequate studies or any evidence that anti-inflammatory diets or other similar strategies reduce the burden of chronic pain.[22]

Naturopathic medicine is considered an alternative to traditional medicine, promoting self-healing and rejecting traditional medicine. Homeopathic medicine is based on the illogic that a substance that causes symptoms of a disease in healthy people will cure a disease in sick people, provided that substance is given in precise, very tiny amounts. The substance is diluted in water or alcohol until only a trace amount or none of it remains. Naturopathy and homeopathy hearken back to snake-oil salespeople, with no evidence of effectiveness in any medical condition.

There are certifying requirements to become a licensed naturopath or homeopath although they vary considerably from state to state. That does not mean that there is any science behind these disciplines. Astrologists can also be licensed. Claims made by naturopaths and homeopaths can be downright dangerous, like this one from a naturopathic publication: "The use of antibiotics should be reserved for those patients who are unresponsive to naturopathic modalities."[23] Fortunately, despite the popularity of complementary medicine, most folks don't try naturopathy or homeopathy. Naturopathy makes up less than 1 percent of visits for complementary health care.[24]

Certain vitamins are often used in patients with chronic pain, but there is almost no evidence that they are effective. Vitamin D may have a role in chronic pain, although studies have been conflicting. Unless you live in a sun-drenched state, it is likely that your blood levels of vitamin D will be below what is considered normal. Some reports have concluded that low serum levels of vitamin D correlate with chronic pain and that vitamin D supplementation mitigates the pain.[25] Other studies have not reached the same conclusion.

The term *nutraceuticals* has been coined to lump together fortified foods, supplements, and specific diets or compounds that have a nutritional and pharmaceutical effect. There is no evidence for their positive impact in chronic pain or any other medical condition. Stephen L. DeFelice, the inventor of that term, stated in 2014, "The quest to demonstrate whether chronic administration, long term diet, long term supplementation, can prevent serious disease like cancer, heart disease, dementia, arthritis, has come to an end."[26] Personalized diets for patients with chronic pain conditions have focused on soy, curcumin, omega-3 fatty acids, and polyphenols, but there is no good evidence that they are useful. Some of these additives and radical diets have been associated with life-threatening liver disease.

Over my lifetime I have tried a number of complementary medicine approaches for pain. I tried to pick those that had some evidence of benefit and that were safe. These included tai chi, yoga, and acupuncture. Each of them gave me some pain relief. I stuck with yoga because it also helped my balance and was easy to incorporate with gentle stretching. I have been taking supplemental vitamin D at the request of my primary care doctor for years. I figure, it can't hurt.

IMPORTANT POINTS ABOUT COMPLEMENTARY MEDICINE AND CHRONIC PAIN

- Yoga, tai chi, and acupuncture can be helpful as adjuncts to traditional medicine in the treatment of chronic pain.
- There is less evidence for the effectiveness of massage, manipulation, chiropractic, and heat or cold, but many people report benefit, and these techniques generally are safe and affordable.
- Vitamins have not been shown to be helpful in chronic pain, except possibly for supplemental vitamin D.
- There is no evidence that naturopathy and homeopathy, specific foods, diets, or supplements decrease chronic pain.

16

MIND-BODY THERAPY

After my brain surgery and seizures, I felt depressed and hopeless. I had always used exercise to help boost my mood, but this time I couldn't force myself to get back to my vigorous routine workouts. The antidepressant Zoloft (sertraline) improved my energy, but I still felt quite helpless until I began weekly counseling. This was not old-fashioned Freudian-style psychotherapy that delves into childhood; rather, it focused on my devastating sense of stress.

Stress can come from anything that overwhelms our capacity to cope, leading to feeling out of control. Physiologically our heart rate increases, breathing becomes shallow, and glucose and oxygen metabolism speed up. The blood supply to our cerebral cortex slows, resulting in mood, sleep, and cognitive disturbances. My therapist and I discussed better ways to cope, and he suggested mindfulness therapy. I was very familiar with mind-body techniques, and we had been using a mindfulness-based stress-reduction program (MBSR) with great success in our patients with chronic pain and fibromyalgia.

Mind-body therapies train people to change maladaptive thoughts, emotions, and behavior, to improve coping strategies, and to increase self-awareness and self-assertiveness. Common thoughts in patients with chronic pain may include, *I am never going to get better*, or *I can't bear this much pain.* These thoughts can become automatic unless they are recognized and reconceptualized. Mindfulness is sometimes defined as the intentional and nonjudgmental awareness of the present moment. Mindfulness teaches you to become more aware of your thoughts, to pause and to step away from your usual automatic stress response. This is often spoken of as a switch from our "doing" mode to a "being" mode. Mind-body techniques quiet the mind, tamping down extraneous noise. It reminds me of professional athletes describing their peak performance as being "in the zone." Their mind switches off and their actions flow without thought or worry.

Meditation is almost always part of mind-body therapy. It may not require the formal practice that most of us picture when we think about meditation. You need not sit motionless for hours in the lotus position. Meditation is any technique that trains one's awareness in order to clear the mind. There are many simple ways to quiet the mind. Many people consider meditation to be simply putting "mind over matter" and that willpower is all you need. We now can point to evidence that meditation and other mind-body therapies achieve pain reduction on a biologic level and, in that sense, work like pain medications.

My associates, a psychiatrist and a clinical nurse specialist, had trained in MBSR with Dr. Jon Kabat-Zinn at the University of Massachusetts Medical Center. Kabat-Zinn had been a molecular biologist but, after spending time in the Far East, became committed to the art and science of meditation. At the University of Massachusetts Medical Center, he developed a very practical and successful MBSR program and published the results of its success in treating hundreds of patients with various illnesses. I read Kabat-Zinn's first book, *Full Catastrophe Living*, in 1990.[1] Kabat-Zinn's MBSR seemed very sensible and easy to learn. I purchased the audiotapes that accompanied that book and began to practice MBSR on my own rather than attending our classes and sitting next to my patients.

Every other day I would set aside one hour and listen to the tapes in a quiet, dark room at home. I had been to a few meditation classes at fancy spas in the past but always found it difficult to not get lost in my thoughts. Kabat-Zinn uses meditation techniques of breathing and guided imagery. Focusing on the breath, you sense the abdomen and chest wall slowly expand as you inhale and then contract as you exhale. While continuing the breathing focus, Kabat-Zinn guides you through a body scan, imaging from the toes up to the head. After thirty minutes of meditation, I flipped the tape over to listen to and perform the simple yoga postures, primarily stretching slowly on a mat, but continuing to incorporate the slow, deep breathing during the stretches. Since then, I have spent at least a few minutes almost daily doing some form of this MBSR and always find it relaxing, calming, and helping with my chronic aches and pains.

In 1993 we published our results using Kabat-Zinn's MBSR program in seventy-seven fibromyalgia patients at our treatment center in Boston.[2] More than 50 percent of our patients showed moderate or marked improvement in pain and function after the ten-week program. Subsequently, a number of studies have demonstrated that MBSR is effective in the treatment of fibromyalgia.[3] An eight-week MBSR program decreased pain and increased function in patients with chronic low back pain and was better than NSAIDs and other analgesics.[4] Based on that study and other similar studies, MBSR is recommended by the American College of Physicians as initial therapy for patients with chronic low back pain. The decreased pain intensity that patients reported after MBSR was found to correlate with changes in brain neural activity, particularly between the insula and anterior cingulate cortex.[5]

Cognitive behavioral therapy (CBT) is another mind-body approach used to treat chronic pain, mood disturbances, and insomnia. CBT uses more directed, problem-focused training than MBSR does. The therapist helps the patient identify maladaptive behavior and then practice strategies to correct that behavior. CBT may be group or individual and often employs techniques such as distraction, imagery, and biofeedback. CBT should be administered by licensed medical professionals, such as mental health therapists, psychologists, or psychiatrists. It is usually performed in a limited number of thirty- to sixty-minute sessions, with a patient expected to practice the skills learned in these sessions and then continue with this practice.

CBT has been found to improve pain, sleep, and mood and to reduce levels of catastrophizing in patients with chronic pain.[6] A CBT program in fibromyalgia that focused on emotional awareness related to psychosocial adversity was particularly effective.[7] CBT was very effective for decreasing the amount of catastrophizing in patients with fibromyalgia.[8] A number of research groups have performed brain imaging before and after CBT, demonstrating that CBT reverses cortical gray matter atrophy and improves functional connectivity in patients with fibromyalgia and other chronic pain conditions.[9]

Both MBSR and CBT have been evaluated in internet-based programs with good results. An MBSR program consisting of twelve online presentations and weekly meditation homework improved symptoms and quality of life in patients with fibromyalgia.[10] CBT, using the online FibroGuide (https://fibroguide.med. umich.edu), developed by the Chronic Pain and Fatigue Research Center at the University of Michigan Medical Center, was effective in fibromyalgia patients. It includes modules for understanding fibromyalgia, communicating, being active, achieving better sleep and relaxation, setting goals, pacing yourself, thinking differently, and setting aside time for yourself. A systematic review of internet-delivered CBT, including seven studies in chronic pain and three in fibromyalgia, found good evidence for its effectiveness.[11] The authors concluded that internet-based CBT shows promise as an alternative to traditional face-to-face therapy.

Biofeedback uses various instruments to provide physiologic information on a stimulus and trains individuals to manipulate their response. One of the most common instruments used to treat chronic pain is an electromyogram (EMG) that measures muscle contraction. An electrode is attached to a specific muscle, and the tension of that muscle is recorded and visualized on a screen. A patient with chronic neck or back pain is trained to relax the offending muscle, receiving positive feedback while observing the fall in muscle tension on the screen. Other techniques have used skin temperature change or heart rate variability. Biofeedback is often incorporated in MBSR and CBT but has also been employed on its own to treat various pain conditions. A systematic review found improved pain and reduced muscle tension in patients with chronic low back pain.[12] Most studies in other pain conditions have been positive, but the reports generally have not been well controlled. Biofeedback employing placebo analgesic conditioning was found to increase pain tolerance in normal individuals.[13]

Hypnosis has also been used to treat various chronic pain conditions, although the evidence for its efficacy is very limited. One problem has been the inability to find a suitable control intervention to compare with hypnosis. Hypnosis does decrease pain perception and increase pain tolerance in a fashion similar to other mind-body therapies.[14]

There are a number of new techniques that rely on mind-body connections to treat chronic pain. The most exciting is noninvasive brain stimulation. This works by applying magnetic or electrical stimulation, externally through the scalp, that can be precisely directed at pain-processing areas in the brain. There are two primary techniques, transcranial direct current stimulation (tDCS) or transcranial electrical stimulation. Both have been extensively studied in chronic pain, especially in fibromyalgia, as well as in mood disturbances.[15] Repetitive tDCS has been shown to produce long-lasting changes in the functional connectivity between pain signaling from the insula to the thalamus.[16]

Such procedures at first seem invasive and conjure up the dark days of electroshock therapy (ECT) in mental illness. But these new techniques are very safe and seem to have no adverse effects on mental function. Currently they are quite costly and usually not covered by insurance. Noninvasive brain stimulation is usually performed at major academic pain centers. However, a recent report described good results from a home-based tDCS program.[17]

Transcutaneous electrical nerve stimulation (TENS) applies electrical current to specific body regions, most often the low back. These electrical currents stimulate or block nerve impulses. TENS has been primarily used to treat chronic low back and neck pain, with some mixed results. It has also been used with significant pain relief in women with fibromyalgia, although a higher electrical current over many sessions was needed.

Based on my personal experience and observing my patients with chronic pain, I am a firm believer in the powerful effects of mind-body therapy. Initially, it was hard for me and many of my patients to believe that such treatment could ever be as helpful as medication. Mind-body therapy should always be used in conjunction with education, exercise, and appropriate medications in the optimal management of chronic pain. Unfortunately, such treatment is often not integrated within most medical practices and may not be easy to find.

IMPORTANT POINTS ABOUT MIND-BODY THERAPY FOR CHRONIC PAIN

* Mind-body therapies, particularly mind-body stress reduction (MBSR) and cognitive behavioral therapy (CBT), are effective in chronic pain management.
* Meditation and various techniques such as biofeedback and imagery are often utilized in mind-body therapy.
* Mind-body therapy has biologic effects on pain processing that are similar to the effects of exercise and various medications. These techniques also help improve mood and sleep disturbances.
* Noninvasive brain magnetic or electrical stimulation has demonstrated efficacy for pain reduction but will require more evaluation before it becomes widely available.
* Mind-body therapies are often not incorporated in standard medical practices but are becoming more available to learn online.

17

FINDING THE RIGHT
HEALTH-CARE TEAM

Effective treatment of chronic pain may not need a whole village but does require an integrated health-care team. This team should include a variety of medical disciplines and health-care professionals. However, the structure of the American medical system makes it difficult to piece together and maintain such an integrated team approach.

Medical care in the United States is organized along disease-specific lines. This works well in cardiology, cancer therapy, orthopedics, and neurology. It does not work in chronic pain. Each medical specialty deals with chronic pain from its own vantage point. A patient with cancer will receive state-of-the-art pain relief from an oncologist. Cardiologists have great expertise in distinguishing chest pain caused by heart disease from that caused by musculoskeletal problems. However, millions of people suffer from chronic pain that does not fall under any one specialist's purview. No medical discipline has claimed ownership of chronic pain as a disease in its own right.

An obvious answer is a pain specialist. Pain medicine is a slowly growing field that was initially dominated by anesthesiology but now includes physical medicine and rehabilitation and other medical specialties. There are only about five thousand pain specialists in the United States. This averages out to one pain specialist for every twenty-nine thousand Americans suffering from chronic pain.[1] In contrast, there are fifty thousand anesthesiologists and thirty-three thousand cardiologists in the United States. Pain specialists can see only a small fraction of our chronic pain population. Pain medicine is a one-year training program, whereas most medical specialties, such as cardiology or rheumatology, are two or three years. Initially pain medicine training was primarily taken by anesthesiologists and focused on interventions for chronic pain, such as nerve and spinal injections and surgical device implantations. These procedures are well reimbursed by medical insurance despite limited evidence for their effectiveness. Most pain medicine training has not emphasized multidisciplinary chronic pain management, which is poorly reimbursed by medical insurance plans.

You and your primary care provider (PCP) make up the nucleus of your health-care team. Your PCP is in charge of making a diagnosis and setting up a treatment plan. This is often straightforward for, say, pneumonia or a bladder infection but almost always complicated with chronic pain. Finding the cause for chronic pain is often difficult, and if the initial evaluation does not provide a clear diagnosis, PCPs usually refer patients to one or more subspecialists. The patient complaining of chronic, widespread pain is appropriately referred to a rheumatologist, the chronic headache patient to a neurologist, and the patient with chronic bowel pain and irritability to a gastroenterologist. The subspecialist may pinpoint the diagnosis, finding a source of organ dysfunction not obvious to the PCP. Early referral to the appropriate subspecialist eliminates needless testing and is time-efficient and cost-effective. The longer the diagnosis takes, the more illness uncertainty and psychosocial stressors adversely affect both patient and physician.

When the specialists do diagnose a specific disease, they will usually take charge. The rheumatologist will take responsibility for treating the pain associated with rheumatoid arthritis. If the rheumatologist decides that the patient does not have rheumatoid arthritis but is suffering from fibromyalgia, the patient is typically sent back to the PCP. If the gastroenterologist excludes the possibility of ulcerative colitis and diagnoses irritable bowel syndrome, the patient is referred back to the PCP. Subspecialists will seldom provide long-term care for patients suffering from common, overlapping chronic pain conditions. There are some fibromyalgia clinics, headache clinics, or pelvic pain clinics at academic medical centers, but they are few and far between.

So chronic pain treatment falls back on the PCP. However, PCPs have neither the time nor the expertise to manage chronic pain. PCPs are overworked and underpaid. There is no time set aside or adequate reimbursement for patient education. With greater attention to electronic medical records and documentation, PCPs often have little face-to-face time with their patients. Most PCPs know that a team approach to chronic pain is ideal but have no way to know which nearby physical therapists, mental health professionals, or complementary health-care practitioners have special interest and skills in treating chronic pain.

An integrated, individualized, multidisciplinary chronic pain management program is the optimal approach for the diagnosis and treatment of chronic pain conditions. Such a multidisciplinary team often includes a pain or rehabilitation specialist, a physical therapist, a social worker, an occupational therapist, a psychologist, and a nurse. The team gets together to arrive at a diagnosis and plan each patient's management. Appointments may involve group education and discussion with providers and patients. In new treatment models, a nurse clinician or a pharmacist may take the lead in most appointments and treatment sessions.

At our fibromyalgia center in Boston, I would evaluate every new patient along with our psychologist and rehabilitation specialist. At that initial assessment, we would conclude the appointment with a one-hour group education session, leaving enough time to answer questions from patients and family members. A similar center in Boston for treating chronic bladder and pelvic pain has included urologists, gynecologists, pelvic floor physical therapists, and pain psychologists. If such multidisciplinary care can be integrated in large primary or subspecialty practices, it can be cost-effective. This has been the model for diabetes care in the United States during the past decade.

In most parts of the country, multidisciplinary chronic pain management groups are not available. In that case, you and your primary health-care provider will need to cobble together a health-care team. Together you may need to shop around for a pain or rehabilitation specialist, a physical therapist, a social worker, an occupational therapist, and a psychologist. You need to ask about their level of interest or expertise in your specific chronic pain problem.

An adequate understanding of your illness is essential to your treatment and critical for a good outcome. As we have discussed, chronic pain is a controversial topic with few absolutes and much conjecture. Some health-care providers, including both PCPs and specialists, are concerned that chronic pain patients are often malingering in an attempt to get disability or financial compensation. Others worry about drug-seeking behavior. For some physicians, chronic pain is a sign of weakness. This is especially true in conditions like fibromyalgia or chronic headaches, where patients look well. Then the severity of their pain is discounted.

Both you and your PCP need to embed the chronic pain diagnosis and management in a biopsychological illness model. Patients with chronic pain that has no structural basis may sense that they are being told, "It is all in your head." They will not feel as if their condition is being taken seriously. More than two-thirds of chronic pain patients express anger toward their health-care providers regarding the confusion in diagnosis and frustrations of trial and error in finding the best treatment or combination of treatments.[2] When patients sense that they are being told their chronic pain has a psychological basis, they tend to sense blame for any failure to recover. This promotes patient embitterment directed at health-care professionals. Women with chronic pain express particular concern about their medical encounters. They describe often feeling rejected and ignored, and seen as whiners or constant complainers. They are most likely to feel as if they are to be blamed for their condition when the chronic pain is linked to any psychological factor.

Counseling with a mental health professional was important in my recovery. Not every chronic pain patient needs to consult with a mental health professional. All chronic pain patients do need to discuss their mood, sleep, and coping mechanisms with their PCP. Those patients with ongoing depression and anxiety should be evaluated and, when appropriate, treated by a mental health professional. The bidirectional interaction of pain and depression warrants that mental health professionals take a significant role in managing chronic pain. However, psychiatrists, psychologists, and therapists often have low confidence and little interest in chronic pain evaluation and management. Making matters more difficult, PCPs seldom can rely on mental health professionals to help them make decisions about a patient's pain or sleep; instead, the mental health professionals will confine their role to treatment of depression or anxiety.

Your family, especially your partner, should be involved in every aspect of your chronic care management. Although it is well known that a supportive family improves health-care outcomes, only 20 percent of adults are accompanied by family members at their chronic care medical appointments.[3] Partners who believe that their loved one's pain is a result of an understandable, organic cause have greater empathy for the patient's difficulty.[4] You and your family all need to buy into the biopsychological illness model.

You need a PCP who is nonjudgmental and listens well. Don't be afraid to switch physicians if you are not satisfied with the level of attention you are receiving. Physician empathy has been linked to patient satisfaction in a variety of chronic pain disorders.[5] Empathy means understanding and placing value on the experiences of another individual. Empathic health care includes a sense of trust, mutual respect, full disclosure, and shared treatment goals. Empathy produces a biologic effect on pain processing, including regulation of the autonomic nervous system and enhanced pain tolerance.[6] Chronic pain patients endorse perceived physician warmth and competence as important components of an empathic relationship.[7]

PCP office visits average fifteen minutes. It is impossible to discuss the many variables and nuances involved in chronic pain care during these brief visits. It makes sense for you and your physician to single out one symptom or situation at a time and focus on that. For example, you may spend one appointment on sleep, another on your concern about the work environment, and yet another on ways to increase your exercise tolerance. Come prepared with a list of your questions and what you have read or heard from others. Frequent visits with your health-care provider foster trust. In patients with chronic pain, increased outpatient health-care engagement decreases the risk of depression and suicide risk. Consistent and frequent longitudinal patient follow-up is critical to the management of chronic pain.

Patients and their health-care professionals need to share in decision-making. Since therapy of chronic pain is largely by trial and error, provider and patient dialogue and flexibility should prevail. Didactic dogma is not productive. Individualized, interdisciplinary care with a biopsychological focus provides the best outcome in chronic pain management but remains out of reach for most Americans in our current health-care system. We need to develop new strategies for interdisciplinary treatment centers, improve self-management of chronic pain, and enable seamless primary care/specialty care collaboration.

IMPORTANT POINTS ABOUT FINDING THE RIGHT HEALTH-CARE TEAM

- Chronic pain care is centered around you and your primary health-care provider (PCP).
- Subspecialists confirm the diagnosis and assume primary responsibility of chronic pain when it is caused by organic disease. Otherwise, your PCP will usually be in charge.

- Chronic pain management should be interdisciplinary, involving physical therapists or rehabilitation specialists, mental health professionals, and pain specialists.
- There are not enough pain specialists in the United States, and their focus is often on procedures.
- Empathy and trust are important in the long-term doctor-patient relationship.
- Involve your family in pain education and management.
- Frequent health-care visits with open discussion are necessary for optimal chronic pain management.

18

YOUR PERSONAL GUIDE TO MANAGING CHRONIC PAIN

GETTING A DIAGNOSIS

There are two distinct issues in the diagnosis of patients with chronic pain. The most obvious is to get an accurate diagnosis. The other is to understand what the diagnosis entails. A few years ago, on the same afternoon, I saw two patients who exemplify these two matters. Both patients, two women around the same age, were referred to me to confirm a presumptive diagnosis of fibromyalgia.

Kate was sixty and had been complaining of stiffness and soreness in her neck, shoulders, upper arms, low back, and thighs for three months. She could barely get out of bed in the morning, and her sleep was interrupted all night by her discomfort. Otherwise she was in good health. The only medication she was taking was one of the statins, Lipitor, for slightly elevated cholesterol, and she had been on that with no adverse side effects for three years. Her PCP, an excellent clinician, told me that he had found no abnormalities on her examination or laboratory testing. This included the acute phase reactants, an ESR and CRP, and the muscle enzyme, CPK.

There were a few clues that fibromyalgia might not have been the correct diagnosis. It is unusual for fibromyalgia to begin at age sixty, and Kate's symptoms began more abruptly than most patients with fibromyalgia. She was complaining more of severe muscle stiffness than widespread pain. I agreed with the PCP that she had no joint swelling, no muscle weakness, and no neurologic abnormalities. On examination, Kate did not have the diffuse muscle tenderness that is characteristic of fibromyalgia. The PCP had ordered the same laboratory tests that I would have. The normal ESR and CRP helped to exclude any inflammatory, systemic disease, and the normal CPK reassured us that she had not developed a muscle disease from taking Lipitor, an uncommon but well-recognized side effect from all statins. I repeated the tests and found that the ESR had gone up, although it was minimally above the normal value. All her other laboratory tests were again normal.

I suspected that Kate might have polymyalgia rheumatica, one of the few causes of these musculoskeletal symptoms that often present with a normal physical examination. Most often the inflammatory blood test markers, ESR and CRP, are very elevated, so that was confusing. However, about 20 percent of patients with polymyalgia rheumatica have normal inflammatory markers on initial laboratory testing. Since those repeat markers had gone up, I decided that polymyalgia rheumatica was the likeliest diagnosis and began Kate on a trial of low-dose prednisone. This usually results in marked resolution of the pain and stiffness within days—exactly what Kate noted. I gradually tapered down and discontinued the prednisone over the next 6 months, with no recurrence of her symptoms.

Most primary care physicians do an excellent initial evaluation when facing a patient with chronic pain. They are attuned to symptoms and signs that signal a potentially dangerous disease, so-called red flags. When confusion arises, specialty referral will almost always resolve the diagnostic dilemma, as happened with Kate. Chronic knee pain from osteoarthritis or back pain from spinal stenosis is seldom misdiagnosed. Whether surgery is the answer can be more complicated and requires the specialist's opinion.

Diagnostic confusion arises when a particular patient's symptoms don't fit the usual pattern. For example, fibromyalgia pain sometimes begins focally, such as in the neck or low back, rather than as characteristic generalized body pain. Some of my chronic pain patients were so concerned with their cognitive symptoms that they kept consulting with neurologists and psychologists. Pain took a back seat to repeated testing for early dementia.

The more timely the diagnosis, the better the outcome. Most chronic pain patients go much too long before an accurate diagnosis is made. Fibromyalgia patients average three years before receiving their diagnosis. This increases our worry and doctor-shopping and wreaks havoc with our psyche, augmenting catastrophizing and other maladaptive pain behaviors.

❋ ❋ ❋

Marion was fifty-seven and had been suffering from widespread pain and exhaustion since she had had a flulike illness when she was forty-six. She told me, "I never got my energy back, and the aching all over my body just got worse. I was always in pain and began taking a lot of ibuprofen, but it didn't help much." Marion's PCP had sent her to an orthopedist, a neurologist, and a rheumatologist, but laboratory testing and X-rays were unrevealing, and no diagnosis was made.

Living in the Northeast, Marion was concerned that she might have Lyme disease and went to a Lyme clinic specialist in Connecticut. Despite never having had the characteristic Lyme rash or positive blood tests for Lyme disease, Marion was told that she had chronic Lyme disease and was treated with daily intravenous antibiotics. Her medical insurance company refused to pay for these treatments, but she continued them for three months without feeling better.

Over the next few years, Marion feverishly sought a cause for her pain and exhaustion. She saw at least ten different specialists. One, a self-styled environmental allergist, told Marion that he suspected toxins in her home were making her sick, hearkening to the so-called sick-building syndrome. All the rugs and carpets were torn out and the ventilation system upgraded, to no effect. Eventually she and her family moved to a new house, but her pain persisted.

Marion's history and physical examination confirmed my suspicion of fibromyalgia. She had been diagnosed with that in the past but did not accept it as a "real disease." Marion believed that if she kept searching, the cause of her symptoms would be found. Eventually she would find answers from a brilliant doctor detective, popularized on television by *House*, which ran on TV from 2004 to 2014. This led to constant doctor-shopping and fragmented care.

I explained to Marion that chronic pain and exhaustion may not conform to simple causal theories of illness. Your primary health-care team and specialist are fully capable of ruling out the diseases that can cause chronic pain. Once those diagnoses are excluded, the chronic pain will fall into one of the overlapping categories personified by fibromyalgia. Marion wanted desperately to find a cause. She fell prey to unscrupulous health-care providers who claim that an infection or allergen cause chronic pain but have no scientific proof to back up those assumptions. It was difficult to convince Marion that her symptoms could be managed without knowing their exact cause and without a disease label.

We discussed the fact that more than 70 percent of chronic pain conditions have no clear physical cause and may best be thought about as illnesses rather than diseases. We label these conditions, based on the primary symptoms, as fibromyalgia, migraine, irritable bowel syndrome, chronic pelvic or bladder pain, and chronic jaw and facial pain. The many alternative explanations and diagnoses she had been given, such as multiple chemical sensitivity syndrome, sick-building syndrome, chronic Epstein-Barr syndrome, and interstitial cystitis, were pseudoscientific labels to satisfy the unrealistic need for medical clarity. The renowned physician and author Lewis Thomas wrote, "The only solid piece of scientific truth about which I feel totally confident is that we are totally ignorant about nature. We do not know how humans work or how they fit in to the enormous, imponderable system of life in which we are embedded as working parts . . . our preoccupation with personal health may be a symptom of copping out, an excuse for running upstairs to recline on a couch, sniffing air for contaminants, spraying the room with deodorants."[1] Accepting the diagnostic uncertainty of chronic pain is essential to a good outcome.

UNDERSTANDING THE MIND-BODY CONNECTION: PERIPHERAL AND CENTRAL PAIN

When I first met Robert, he could barely get himself out of the waiting-room chair. He hobbled into my office, using a cane for support. He was a divorced forty-five-year-old man who looked somewhat disheveled and was in obvious pain. Robert had worked in a number of jobs, mainly in manual labor, until at age thirty-seven his back "went out" after lifting some heavy boxes. He was referred to a doctor from his company and was treated with two weeks of bed rest and oxycodone. The pain continued, and he saw a chiropractor recommended by some friends. Robert told me, "[After the chiropractor] cracked my back, I couldn't even bend over to tie my shoes. The pain was excruciating, and I essentially became an invalid."

An orthopedist examined Robert, and an MRI revealed disk degeneration. The orthopedist recommended a course of physical therapy, increased the dose of oxycodone, and added pregabalin to be taken at bedtime. Over the next six months there was no improvement, the pain was continuous, and Robert filed for disability insurance. During the next few years Robert battled with the insurance company and finally received workers' compensation, but it was so meager that he had to borrow money from his parents.

He consulted with another back surgeon, who suggested that Robert undergo surgery to remove the degenerative disk. Robert decided to try physical therapy one more time, but after a few

sessions without any pain relief, he had the back surgery. Unfortunately, things went from bad to worse.

At his initial visit Robert described the back pain as "ten out of
ten." During the prior few years, he had also had constant pain in
his neck and upper back. The back pain also had spread to his legs,
but he did not describe the neurologic symptoms characteristic of
sciatica, and there were no motor or sensory abnormalities.

Robert described his daily routine as a bed-to-chair existence.
Most days he tried to take a walk, but for the past year he had
needed a cane, even when walking a few blocks. He admitted to
being discouraged, depressed, and angry, both at his doctors and
his former employer, telling me, "No one believes how much pain
I have. You have no idea what I am going through."

Robert's struggle with chronic back pain is representative of an
all-too-familiar story. He held fast to the notion that the back pain
was caused by physical damage to his lower back. Injuries should
heal, so why hadn't his?

Robert's treatment followed the outdated causal theories of
chronic pain. If this was an injury, it was logical to stay in bed for a
few weeks. We now know that bed rest makes everything worse
and appropriate movement, stretching, and strengthening are necessary for recovery. Manipulation made sense, since he was told
his lower back was out of alignment. There is seldom any misalignment in patients with lower back pain unless severe spinal curva-
ture or scoliosis is present. Finally, surgery gave Robert the
chance to remove the source of his pain. He would get rid of the
degenerated disk and then finally get rid of the pain. No one
cautioned Robert that by age forty almost everybody has disk degeneration and there is no link between chronic low back pain
with disk degeneration. Fortunately, disk removal for chronic low
back pain is no longer routinely offered to patients with chronic
low back pain, but not long ago, when Robert consulted with a
back surgeon, it was still commonplace.

I reinforced the biopsychological model of chronic pain and the
research demonstrating that a well-defined, physical cause of
chronic low back is found in less than 10 percent of cases.[2] Rob-

ert's widespread pain, now involving his neck, shoulders, upper back, and legs, was consistent with fibromyalgia, and I explained that persistent focal pain will often morph into a more generalized pain. We went over the science behind the key role of central nervous system hypersensitivity.

Robert had been taking opioids daily for eight years. Each time he attempted to decrease the dose, his pain increased. He told me, "Some of my doctors think I'm a junkie and refuse to treat me. They are the ones that got me into this mess, and now they want to get rid of me." Chronic low back pain is the most common medical diagnosis listed for prescribing opioids in the United States, despite the lack of evidence for their efficacy. Robert and I spent the first few sessions discussing this, since he was most concerned that I would be another in the long line of physicians accusing him of seeking drugs. There is a stigma associated with opioid use, suggesting weak character.

I told Robert he undoubtedly was opioid-dependent but that that was a normal physiologic response to long-term opioid use. He was not a drug addict. He agreed to consult with our pain specialist, who first switched Robert to a buprenorphine/naloxone combination. The pain specialist then very slowly began to wean him off opioids and to substitute with a combination of other medications. This needed to be done carefully, because abrupt tapering of opioids would lead to greater pain and promote mistrust in the doctor-patient relationship.

Robert was most cynical about joining our mind-body/stress reduction program, and I was equally skeptical that he would benefit from it. His background and beliefs did not seem to be conducive to such an approach to chronic pain. Already angry about losing his job, going through litigation, lacking much family support, he seemed to me an unlikely candidate for self-reflection. Since he was a heavy smoker and had taken opioids for years, also risk factors for poor outcome in patients with chronic pain, I doubted that Robert would be willing to make major lifestyle changes. How wrong I was.

Within a few sessions, he became an active contributor in our MBSR program. Robert told me, "It was helpful to hear that others had gone through the same problems. We could share our frustration without feeling like we were failures." He even stuck with breathing exercises and body scan techniques, noting how they helped him relax and drew attention away from his pain.

Robert has worked diligently with one of our physical therapists. Initially this consisted of massage and deep-tissue work, with short periods of time on a stationary bike. Gradually he began taking longer walks without needing a cane. With encouragement from the physical therapist, he joined a tai chi class and became a regular member. He was proud of what he could do with these added movements and postures and felt more empowered.

After watching Robert's progress over the past five years, I am encouraged that even in situations that look hopeless to both patient and physician, chronic pain can be managed, if not cured. Robert still has a lot of back pain, although the more generalized pain has abated. He consulted with a new back surgeon, and a recent lumbar MRI revealed further disc degeneration and moderate spinal stenosis. Robert asked me what I thought about the surgeon's recommendation that he have a lumbar fusion. Over the course of our five years together, I had discussed my own back pain and Robert knew that I had had good results from spinal stenosis surgery. If he had asked me this same question seven years earlier, I would have dissuaded him from undergoing the disk surgery. Even then, disk removal to cure chronic low back pain was overhyped and underresearched. At that time, Robert also had all the signs and symptoms of severe fibromyalgia, in addition to his chronic low back pain.

My colleague Dr. Dan Clauw and his collaborators at the University of Michigan have reported that the severity of fibromyalgia symptoms correlates well with outcomes after major surgery.[3] Those patients with more pain, exhaustion, and mood and sleep disturbances, even if they had never been diagnosed with fibromyalgia, had poorer results from surgery and required more postoperative opioids. Robert currently was free of widespread pain, and his sleep and mood had dramatically improved. Still, the decision about undergoing further surgery was not easy.

Even with the recognition that central sensitization is a driving force behind chronic pain, peripheral pain generators can't be ignored. Low back pain often improves with heat, massage, manipulation, injections, and acupuncture. How you lift, sit, and work, so-called ergonomics, are important in chronic back and neck pain.

In patients with severe knee or hip osteoarthritis, successful joint replacement surgery not only eliminates the knee or hip pain but also improves concurrent widespread pain. After contemplating this information, Robert decided to have the spinal stenosis surgery. At his last visit Robert told me that his back pain was much improved and that he was attending night classes and hoped to learn a new trade and go back to work.

☼ ☼ ☼

I first met Sarah when she was fifty. She had a history of chronic headaches since childhood. They were typical of tension headaches, although once a year she would have a severe attack of migraine. At age forty she began experiencing back and neck pain. Over the next few years, the pain became more generalized, and she also began having pelvic pain. Sarah's sleep was constantly interrupted by pain or the urge to void. She then began having difficulty falling asleep and was constantly exhausted.

Sarah had been diagnosed with postpartum depression after the birth of her second daughter fifteen years ago. She was treated with an antidepressant and counseling for about one year with no subsequent depression. She described herself as a worrier but had no symptoms to suggest major anxiety. Since her pain began, she had become increasingly concerned that she was no longer functioning adequately as a mother and a wife. As an example, she tearfully mentioned that she had lost all interest in sexual relations with her husband. Sarah said, "I can't focus on anything except the pain."

Sarah's husband accompanied her to the initial appointment and has been with her at each subsequent office visit. I have found him to be very supportive and never judgmental. I explained to them that I was quite convinced that Sarah had fibromyalgia and told them what that entailed. They had read about fibromyalgia, and Sarah expressed two major concerns: "Was it all in my head?" and "Was there any effective treatment?"

We tackled the first question by reviewing the biopsychological model that is the framework for every chronic pain disorder. I discussed the evidence that chronic pain alters brain signaling, resulting in central nervous system hypersensitivity—like the amplifier on a sound machine being constantly cranked up. Thoughts and emotions theoretically can increase or decrease this pain hypersensitivity. With this background, we delved into Sarah's prior psychosocial history.

After meeting with Sarah a few times, I felt confident that she was not experiencing major depression and did not need a formal psychiatric diagnostic interview. She was experiencing anxiety about her persistent pain and inability to get a good night's sleep. We discussed the negative impact of her illness ruminations and ways to counter that. She began attending our Mind-Body Stress Reduction program. After a few months, Sarah told me that she was able to let go of negative emotions and felt in much better control of the pain.

EXERCISE, SLEEP

Sarah had always been very active and was exercising regularly until her neck and back pain became so prominent ten years earlier. Since then, Sarah had been quite sedentary, other than doing household chores and driving her girls to their activities. She gained forty pounds over the past few years.

As her sleep became more erratic, Sarah began lying down and attempting to nap during the day. With her weight gain, I was concerned that Sarah might have developed sleep apnea, and her husband reported that she did snore. I sent her to a sleep specialist, who found no evidence for sleep apnea. Then I began Sarah on a small amount of Elavil (amitriptyline) at bedtime, and her sleep quickly improved. After a few visits, she was still complaining of exhaustion, so I added a small amount of Zoloft (sertraline) to be taken in the morning. With those two medications, Sarah's energy perked up and she felt able to begin some walking.

We discussed the short-term goal of being less sedentary and the long-range goals of weight reduction and a general physical fitness program. Sarah began to go out for daily walks, and within a few months, she and her husband joined a health club. They started with water exercise classes and gradually added some resistance exercise training. I reviewed the lack of evidence that specific foods or radical diets caused chronic pain. I encouraged her to follow a healthy diet but to stop looking for answers to her pain in what she was eating. Over the next year Sarah lost most of the forty pounds that she had gained and was exercising regularly at least four times weekly.

We treated the tension headaches with massage and myofascial tissue work. Our rehabilitation specialist began Sarah on a series of acupuncture treatments, both designed to help her headaches and lessen the pelvic and bladder pain. She also began pelvic strengthening, called Kegel exercises, and over the next year began doing yoga classes. For the past ten years, Sarah had been fearful that excess movement or exercise would aggravate her pain. When that fear of movement dissipated, her pain lessened, and her functioning greatly improved.

Sarah followed sleep hygiene recommendations that included going to bed at the same time each night and confining her naps to a brief power nap in the early afternoon. When we have insomnia, we typically try to catch up on our sleep deprivation by going to bed much earlier. That doesn't work, and it contributes to sleep anxiety. Sarah was staying awake for hours, worrying that she would not be able to function without adequate sleep. The MBSR program taught her ways to deal with this sleep anxiety, and she began using imagery or other body scans to help her fall asleep.

Modifiable lifestyle factors determine the adequacy of our sleep. Sleep disturbances are a major contributor to chronic pain. The weight loss and exercise were major contributors to her improved sleep.

THE DOCTOR-PATIENT RELATIONSHIP

Marion had been unhappy with the many physicians she had seen as she sought answers for her chronic pain. Her story indicated that the breakdown in her past doctor-patient relationships fell both on her shoulders and those of her physicians. As we have discussed, most clinicians consider patients with chronic pain to be the most difficult to manage.[4] Chronic pain care is described by physicians as frustrating, time-consuming, complicated, and likely to fail.[5]

Some of Marion's physicians probably thought that her multiple pain complaints were exaggerated or even hypochondriacal. Some physicians likely thought the same thing about Robert, who was accused of being a "drug seeker." Physicians uniformly rate chronic pain patients' pain levels as less severe than do the patients themselves.

When chronic pain patients are like Marion and disagree with their physicians about the cause of their pain, they are dissatisfied with their care.

You need to feel that your physicians are concerned about you and your level of pain, that they listen nonjudgmentally. When chronic pain patients sense that their pain is not taken seriously, they report low levels of confidence in diagnostic and treatment plans, and feelings of alienation.[6] Frequent contact with health-care providers is vital to optimal management of chronic pain. And optimal management can be most accessible with a team approach to your care, where your primary physician shares responsibility with various other health-care providers.

You also need to take charge of your care. This requires active participation. At first glance, Marion seemed to be very active, seeking multiple consultations from all sorts of specialists. In fact, she was passive-aggressive, insisting on an answer without a willingness to change her health-care attitudes and lifestyle.

Most physicians have moved away from a "doctor knows best" attitude to a collaborative care model. That is crucial in chronic pain management. A number of studies have demonstrated that more active patient self-management is helpful in chronic pain and can be taught.[7] Sarah and Robert have both taken an active role in managing their chronic pain. Self-management in patients with chronic pain must include patient education about physical activity, exercise, pacing, sleep, and the role of stress and mood.

TREATMENT AND OUTCOME

The cornerstone of chronic pain management is patient and family education. Before embarking on a specific therapy, you must understand chronic pain as a disease, played out within a bio-psychological illness framework. You and your primary physician should focus on risk factors for chronic pain that can be modified, such as lack of exercise, obesity, cigarette smoking, opioid misuse, stress, and excess illness worry. Robert and Sarah bought into this illness model.

Robert was taken aback when I suggested that medication often takes a back seat to nonpharmacologic management of chronic pain. We all are accustomed to thinking that pills are the best treatment for any illness. That is certainly true for an infection. In the treatment of chronic pain, medications are best utilized in combination with many other treatment modalities. Robert and Sarah were open to trying things like yoga, tai chi, meditation, and acupuncture.

Both were able to access an integrated, multidisciplinary pain management program. They both have worked diligently with a team of health-care providers, including some who are experts in activity and exercise and others who are experts in how to better cope with chronic illness and stress. Such programs are usually not part of primary care practice. Hopefully, you and your PCP can locate such an integrated program or find various providers to form your own. You should make use of educational and treatment tools available on the internet. As discussed in chapter 3, this may include online information, telemedicine, and patient support groups. For example, a telephone-delivered collaborative care management program called Stepped Care to Optimize Pain care Effectiveness (SCOPE) was found to significantly reduce pain and improve mood and function in patients with chronic, widespread pain.[8]

Sarah asked me whether I thought that she should return to work. We discussed potential workplace stressors, which had never seemed too great for her until her pain became intolerable. I told her that research studies found that women who continued to work despite having fibromyalgia had much better health outcomes than those who stopped working.[9]

Over the past few years Sarah and Robert have both been doing well. Both get occasional exacerbations of their chronic pain. Sarah often attributes these flare-ups to increases in her stress levels. Stress of any type heightens pain and makes treatment more difficult. I have talked to both Sarah and Robert about expected symptom flare-ups in their chronic pain. They are keeping logs noting potential factors in these flare-ups and ways to go about dealing with those.

Both Sarah and Robert were concerned with reports that chronic pain leads to dementia and early death. I reassured them that there is no evidence of mental decline or premature death in patients who respond well to chronic pain management. Any increased mortality in patients with chronic pain is related to severe depression and an increase in suicide rates.

Sarah was interested in seeing how she would do without the two medications, so I gradually tapered one and then the other. However, after a few weeks her pain increased, and her sleep became more erratic, so we reinstituted the medications, with good results. Although she does not routinely practice mind-body techniques, Sarah finds ways to relax and tune out excess worry.

Sarah continues to exercise regularly and has kept her weight stable.

Sarah and Robert have each made remarkable progress in their battles with chronic pain. There were common aspects to their road to recovery. They included an acceptance of illness uncertainty and an understanding of the mind-body interaction. Some soul-searching may be needed, particularly with regard to our emotional response to chronic pain. Emotions don't cause pain, but they aggravate and perpetuate chronic pain. As I stated earlier, my bouts of pain and depression were associated with feelings of helplessness and hopelessness.

Sarah and Robert have learned how to separate medical fact from fiction, rejecting the false claims that there was a magic potion. Unfortunately, Marion could never stop searching for the cause, for her holy grail. She held fast to having to find a disease diagnosis if she was ever going to conquer her pain. Without knowing the cause, her pain would never be cured. Sarah and Robert accepted the reality that chronic pain is seldom cured but can be managed.

Chronic pain is the most prevalent, disabling, and expensive health condition in the United States, affecting more than one hundred million people with an annual cost of $640 million.[10] Despite this, there has been relatively little recent research or progress made on chronic pain management. We have a long way to go, particularly in developing new medications that effectively reduce pain. Our American opioid crisis is a stark reminder of what can happen when greed overtakes the rational need for better and safer analgesics.

The American Pain Society identified five broad goals to stem the epidemic of chronic pain:[11]

1. Develop novel pain treatments that enhance clinically meaningful pain relief and functional improvement with acceptable adverse effects.
2. Expedite progress toward the prevention, diagnosis, and management of chronic pain conditions.

3. Optimize the use of and access to currently available treatments that are known to be effective.
4. Understand the impact of health policies and systems on pain treatment.
5. Improve pain management through education research.

This book has highlighted the common nature of all types of chronic pain. Historically considered to be distinct disorders, chronic pain conditions share clinical and epidemiologic features. Pathophysiologically, altered neurologic mechanisms lead to sensory hyperirritability, which in turn perpetuates the chronicity of pain as well as chronic mood and sleep disturbances.

This book is dedicated to the thousands of my patients and colleagues who have been part of my personal and professional journey to better understand and treat chronic pain. Chronic pain is not easy to define, measure, or treat. Elaine Scarry summed it up nicely when she wrote, "Pain comes . . . into our midst as at once that which cannot be denied and that which cannot be confirmed."[12] Hopefully this book has provided some understanding of the nature of chronic pain and a pathway to its optimal treatment.

IMPORTANT POINTS ABOUT OPTIMAL CHRONIC PAIN MANAGEMENT

- Diagnosis and treatment recommendations should come from your PCP and, when necessary, should involve specialist confirmation and further guidance.
- A timely diagnosis and a timely treatment plan are important.
- Most often, there is no single cause of chronic pain.
- Chronic pain diagnosis and treatment must be framed within a biopsychological illness model.
- Exercise is the most cost-effective approach to treating chronic pain and coexisting sleep and mood disturbances.

- Medications, used judiciously, can be helpful, but chronic opioids should be avoided.
- Mind-body therapy should be part of an integrated, multidisciplinary chronic pain management program.
- You must be an active participant in all aspects of your care.

NOTES

1. CHRONIC PAIN

1. James Dahlhamer et al., "Prevalence of Chronic Pain and High-Impact Chronic Pain among Adults: United States, 2016," *Morbidity and Mortality Weekly Report* 67, no. 36 (September 14, 2018): 1001–6. doi:10.15585/mmwr.mm6736a2.

2. Institute of Medicine Committee on Advancing Pain Research, Care, and Education, *Relieving Pain in America: A Blueprint for Transforming Prevention, Care, Education, and Research* (Washington, DC: National Academies Press, 2011).

3. Ibid.

4. Ibid.

5. Ibid.

6. Walter F. Stewart et al., "Lost Productive Time and Cost Due to Common Pain Conditions in the US Workforce," *Journal of the American Medical Association* 290 (2003): 2443–54.

7. Caitlin Murray et al., "Long-Term Impact of Adolescent Chronic Pain on Young Adult Educational, Vocational, and Social Outcomes," *Pain* (October 21, 2019), doi:10.1097/j.pain.0000000000001732.

8. Institute of Medicine Committee, *Relieving Pain in America*.

9. Thomas A. Coffelt, Benjamin D. Bauer, and Aaron E. Carroll, "Inpatient Characteristics of the Child Admitted with Chronic Pain," *Pediatrics* 132, no. 2 (2013): e422.

10. Janet K. Freburger et al., "The Rising Prevalence of Chronic Low Back Pain," *Archives of Internal Medicine* 169 (2009): 251–58.

11. Institute of Medicine Committee, *Relieving Pain in America.*

12. Stanley Tweyman, *René Descartes: Meditations on First Philosophy in Focus* (New York: Routledge, 1993), 34–40.

13. Blair Smith et al., "The IASP Classification of Chronic Pain for ICD-11: Applicability in Primary Care," *Pain* 160 (2019): 83–87.

14. Don L. Goldenberg, "Fibromyalgia: Why Such Controversy?" *Annals of Rheumatic Diseases* 54 (1995): 3–5.

15. Kassondra L. Collins et al., "A Review of Current Theories and Treatments for Phantom Limb Pain," *Journal of Clinical Investigation* 128 (2018): 2168–76.

16. Jamila Andoh et al., "Neural Correlates of Evoked Phantom Limb Sensations," *Biological Psychology* 126 (2017): 89–97.

17. Institute of Medicine Committee, *Relieving Pain in America.*

18. Smith et al., "The IASP Classification of Chronic Pain for ICD-11."

2. MIND AND/OR BODY

1. Hans Christian Andersen, *The Princess and the Pea* (Copenhagen: C. A. Reitzel, 1835).

2. UnCheol Lee et al., "Functional Brain Network Mechanism of Hypersensitivity in Chronic Pain," *Scientific Reports* 8 (2018): 243–66.

3. Ibid.

4. Tor D. Wager et al., "An fMRI-Based Neurologic Signature of Physical Pain," *New England Journal of Medicine* 368 (2013): 1388–97.

5. Marina Lopez-Sola et al., "Towards a Neurophysiological Signature for Fibromyalgia," *Pain* 158 (2017): 34–47.

6. Matthew J. Bair et al., "Depression and Pain Comorbidity: A Literature Review," *Archives of Internal Medicine* 163 (2003): 2433–45.

7. Maurice M. Ohayon and Alan F. Schatzberg, "Chronic Pain and Major Depressive Disorder in the General Population," *Journal of Psychiatric Research* 44 (2010): 454–61.

8. John McBeth et al., "Sleep Disturbances and Chronic Widespread Pain," *Current Rheumatology Reports* 17 (2015): 469–86.

9. Ibid.

10. Xaver Fuchs, Herta Flor, and Robin Bekrater-Bodmann, "Psychological Factors Associated with Phantom Limb Pain: A Review of Recent Findings," *Pain Research Management* 2018, no. 5080123 (June 21, 2018), doi:10.1155/2018/5080123.

11. John Haygarth, *Of the Imagination, as a Cause and as a Cure of Disorders of the Body, Exemplified by Fictitious Tractors, and Epidemical Convulsions* (Bath, England: Crutwell, 1801).

12. Donald D. Price, Damien G. Finniss, and Fabrizio Benedetti, "A Comprehensive Review of the Placebo Effect: Recent Advances and Current Thought," *Annual Review of Psychology* 59 (2008): 565–90.

13. Janie Luana Colloca Damien, Carmen-Édith Bellei-Rodriguez, and Serge Marchand, "Pain Modulation: From Conditioned Pain Modulation to Placebo and Nocebo Effects in Experimental and Clinical Pain," *International Review of Neurobiology* 139 (2018): 255–96.

14. Ibid.

15. Gareth T. Jones et al., "Role of Road Traffic Accidents and Other Traumatic Events in the Onset of Chronic Widespread Pain: Results from a Population-Based Prospective Study," *Arthritis Care & Research* 63 (2011): 696–701.

3. NATURE OR NURTURE, AND THE GENDER GAP

1. James J. Cox et al., "An SCN9A Channelopathy Causes Congenital Inability to Experience Pain," *Nature* 444 (2006): 894–98.

2. Justin Heckert, "The Hazards of Growing Up Painlessly," *New York Times*, November 15, 2012.

3. Abdella M. Habib et al., "Microdeletion in a FAAH Pseudogene Identified in a Patient with High Anandamide Concentrations and Pain Insensitivity," *British Journal of Anaesthesia* 123 (2019): 249–53.

4. Katerina Zorina-Lichtenwalter et al., "Genetic Predictors of Human Chronic Pain Conditions," *Neuroscience* 338 (2016): 36–62.

5. Ibid.

6. Edwin Aroke et al., "Could Epigenetics Help Explain Racial Disparities in Chronic Pain?" *Journal of Pain Research* 12 (2019): 701–10.

7. Jasmine I. Kerr and Andrea Burri, "Genetic and Epigenetic Epidemiology of Chronic Widespread Pain," *Journal of Pain Research* 10 (2017): 2021–29.

8. Institute of Medicine Committee, *Relieving Pain in America*.

9. Ingunn Mundal et al., "Psychosocial Factors and Risk of Chronic Widespread Pain: An 11-Year Follow-Up Study—The HUNT Study," *Pain* 155 (2014): 1555–61.

10. Aleksi Varinen et al., "The Relationship between Childhood Adversities and Fibromyalgia in the General Population," *Journal of Psychosomatic Research* 99 (2017): 137–42.

11. Winfried Häuser et al., "Posttraumatic Stress Disorder in Fibromyalgia Syndrome: Prevalence, Temporal Relationship between Posttraumatic Stress and Fibromyalgia Symptoms, and Impact on Clinical Outcome," *Pain* 154 (2013): 1216–23.

12. John McBeth et al., "Moderation of Psychosocial Risk Factors through Dysfunction of the Hypothalamic-Pituitary-Adrenal Stress Axis in the Onset of Chronic Widespread Musculoskeletal Pain: Findings of a Population-Based Prospective Cohort Study," *Arthritis Rheumatology* 56 (2007): 360–71.

13. Senthil Packiasabapathy and Senthilkumar Sadhasivam, "Gender, Genetics, and Analgesia: Understanding the Differences in Response to Pain Relief," *Journal of Pain Research* 11 (2018): 2729–39.

14. Ru-Rong Ji et al., "Neuroinflammation and Central Sensitization in Chronic and Widespread Pain," *Anesthesiology* 129 (2018): 343–66.

15. Packiasabapathy and Sadhasivam, "Gender, Genetics, and Analgesia."

16. Susan E. Abbey and Paul E. Garfinkel, "Neurasthenia and Chronic Fatigue Syndrome: The Role of Culture in the Making of a Diagnosis," *American Journal of Psychiatry* 148 (1991): 1638–46.

17. Virginia Woolf, "On Being Ill," in *The Criterion*, by T. S. Eliot (London: Hogarth Press, 1926).

18. Melvin Blanchard et al., "Medical Correlates of Chronic Multisymptom Illness in Gulf War Veterans," *American Journal of Medicine* 132 (2019): 510–18.

19. Pierluca Coiro and Daniela D. Pollak, "Sex and Gender Bias in the Experimental Neurosciences," *Translational Psychiatry* 9 (2019): 90–98.

4. PAIN EDUCATION AND MISINFORMATION

1. Robert W. Gereau IV et al., "A Pain Research Agenda for the 21st Century," *Journal of Pain* 15 (2014): 1203–14.

2. Ibid.

3. R. J. W. Cline and K. M. Haynes, "Consumer Health Information Seeking on the Internet: The State of the Art," *Health Education Research* 16 (2001): 671–92.

4. Ibid.

5. William M. Silberg, George D. Lundberg, and Robert A. Musacchio, "Assessing, Controlling, and Assuring the Quality of Medical Information on the Internet," *Journal of the American Medical Association* 277 (1997): 1244–45.

6. Mike Benigeri and Pierre Pluye, "Shortcomings of Health Information on the Internet," *Health Promotion International* 18 (2003): 381–86.

7. Faith McLellan, "'Like Hunger, Like Thirst': Patients, Journals, and the Internet," *Lancet* 352 Supplement 2 (1999): 39–43.

8. Cline and Haynes, "Consumer Health Information Seeking on the Internet."

9. Gunther Eysenbach, John Powell, and Oliver Kuss, "Empirical Studies Assessing the Quality of Health Information for Consumers on the World Wide Web: A Systematic Review," *Journal of the American Medical Association* 287 (2002): 2691–700.

10. Lubna Daraz et al., "The Quality of Websites Addressing Fibromyalgia: An Assessment of Quality and Readability Using Standardised Tools," *British Medical Journal Open* 1, no. 1 (2011): e000152.

11. Laura Butler and Nadine Foster, "Back Pain Online: A Cross-Sectional Survey of the Quality of Web-Based Information on Low Back Pain," *Spine* 28 (2003): 395–401.

12. Benigeri and Pluye, "Shortcomings of Health Information."

13. Julie M. Donohue, Marisa Cevasco, and Meredith B. Rosenthal, "A Decade of Direct-to-Consumer Advertising of Prescription Drugs," *New England Journal of Medicine* 357 (2007): 673–81.

14. Ibid.

15. Joseph Dumit, "Pharmaceutical Witnessing: Drugs for Life in an Era of Direct-to-Consumer Advertising," in *The Pharmaceutical Studies*

Reader, ed. Sergio Sismondo and Jeremy A. Greene (Manchester, UK: Wiley Blackwell, 2015).

16. Tabetha K. Violet, "Constructing the Gendered Risk of Illness in Lyrica Ads for Fibromyalgia: Fear of Isolation as a Motivating Narrative for Consumer Demand," *Journal of Medical Humanities*, https://doi.org/10.1007/s10912-019-09575-9.

17. Ibid.

18. Lina Mezei and Beth B. Murinson, "Pain Education in North American Medical Schools," *Journal of Pain* 12 (2011): 1199–208.

19. Gereau et al., "A Pain Research Agenda."

20. Ibid.

21. Adam Hirsh et al., "Preferences, Experience, and Attitudes in the Management of Chronic Pain and Depression: A Comparison of Physicians and Medical Students," *Clinical Journal of Pain* 30 (2014): 766–84.

22. Donohue, Cevasco, and Rosenthal, "A Decade of Direct-to-Consumer Advertising."

23. Institute of Medicine, *Relieving Pain in America*.

5. FIBROMYALGIA

1. Harvey Moldofsky et al., "Musculoskeletal Symptoms and Non-REM Sleep Disturbance in Patients with 'Fibrositis Syndrome' and Healthy Subjects," *Psychosomatic Medicine* 37 (1975): 341–51.

2. McBeth et al., "Sleep Disturbances and Chronic Widespread Pain."

3. Ibid.

4. Adam J. Krause et al., "The Pain of Sleep Loss: A Brain Characterization in Humans," *Journal of Neuroscience* 39 (2019): 2291–300.

5. Michael D. Reynolds, "The Development of the Concept of Fibrositis," *Journal of History of Medical Allied Sciences* 38 (1983): 7–13.

6. Lesley M. Arnold et al., "Family Study of Fibromyalgia," *Arthritis Rheumatology* 50 (2004): 944–52.

7. Don L. Goldenberg and Hartej S. Sandhu, "Fibromyalgia and Post-Traumatic Stress Disorder," *Seminars in Arthritis and Rheumatism* 32 (2002): 1–2.

8. James Robinson et al., "Determination of Fibromyalgia Syndrome after Whiplash Injuries: Methodologic Issues," *Pain* 152 (2011): 1311–16.

9. Kathleen Dorado et al., "Interactive Effects of Pain Catastrophizing and Mindfulness on Pain Intensity in Women with Fibromyalgia," *Health Psychology Open* 5, no. 2 (October 22, 2018), doi:10.1177/2055102918807406.

10. Don L. Goldenberg, "Fibromyalgia Syndrome a Decade Later: What Have We Learned?" *Archives of Internal Medicine* 159 (1999): 777–85.

11. Kathleen A. Sluka and Daniel J. Clauw, "Neurobiology of Fibromyalgia and Chronic Widespread Pain," *Neuroscience* 338 (2016): 114–29.

12. Ibid.

13. Goldenberg, "Fibromyalgia: Why Such Controversy?"

14. Frederick Wolfe et al., "The American College of Rheumatology 1990 Criteria for the Classification of Fibromyalgia," *Arthritis Rheumatology* 33 (1990): 160–72.

15. Don L. Goldenberg, "Fibromyalgia: To Diagnose or Not. Is That Still the Question?" *Journal of Rheumatology* 31, no. 4 (May 2004): 633–35.

16. Goldenberg, "Fibromyalgia Syndrome a Decade Later."

17. Omer Gendelman et al., "Time to Diagnosis of Fibromyalgia and Factors Associated with Delayed Diagnosis in Primary Care," *Best Practice & Research Clinical Rheumatology* 32 (2018): 489–99.

18. Victoria Silverwood et al., "'If It's a Medical Issue I Would Have Covered It by Now': Learning about Fibromyalgia through the Hidden Curriculum: A Qualitative Study," *BMC Medical Education* 17 (2017): 160–96.

19. Katie Scott, "Lady Gaga Cancels Rio Performance after Being Hospitalized for 'Severe Physical Pain,'" Global News, September 15, 2017, https://globalnews.ca/news/3747264/lady-gaga-severe-pain.

20. *Gaga: Five Foot Two* (Netflix, 2017).

21. Ibid.

22. Ibid.

23. Ibid.

6. MIGRAINE

1. Richard B. Lipton et al., "Migraine Prevalence, Disease Burden, and the Need for Preventive Therapy," *Neurology* 68 (2007): 343–49.

2. Oliver Sacks, *Migraine*, rev. and exp. (New York: Vintage Books, 1999).

3. Charles Carrington, *Rudyard Kipling: His Life and Work* (London: Macmillan, 1955).

4. Klaus Podoll and Derek Robinson, "Lewis Carroll's Migraine Experiences," *Lancet* 353 (1999): 1366.

5. Ibid.

6. Lipton et al., "Migraine Prevalence, Disease Burden."

7. Ibid.

8. Walter Alvarez, "The Migrainous Personality and Constitution," *American Journal of the Medical Sciences* 213 (1947): 1–8.

9. Sacks, *Migraine*.

10. George Beard, *A Practical Treatise on Nervous Exhaustion* (New York: W. Wood, 1880).

11. Quoted in Sacks, *Migraine*.

12. Ibid.

13. Vincent T. Martin and Brinder Vij, "Diet and Headache: Part 1," *Headache* 56, no. 9 (October 2016): 1543–52.

14. Ibid.

15. Lee B. Peterlin et al., "Sex Matters: Evaluating Sex and Gender in Migraine and Headache Research," *Headache* 51 (2011): 839–42.

16. Anne E. MacGregor, Jason D. Rosenberg, and Tobias Kurth, "Sex-Related Differences in Epidemiological and Clinic-Based Headache Studies," *Headache* 51 (2011): 843–59.

17. Padhraig Gormley et al., "Migraine Genetics: From Genome-Wide Association Studies to Translational Insights," *Genome Medicine* 8 (2016): 86. doi:10.1186/s13073-016-0346-4.

18. Zachary F. Gerring et al., "Genome-Wide DNA Methylation Profiling in Whole Blood Reveals Epigenetic Signatures Associated with Migraine," *BMC Genomics* 19 (2018): 69–79.

19. William R. Gowers, *The Border-Land of Epilepsy* (London: Churchill, 1907).

20. Sacks, *Migraine*.

21. Daniela Pietrobon and Michael A. Moskowitz, "Chaos and Commotion in the Wake of Cortical Spreading Depression and Spreading Depolarizations," *Nature Reviews Neuroscience* 15 (2014): 379–93.

22. Julio A. Yanes, "Toward a Multimodal Framework of Brainstem Pain-Modulation Circuits in Migraine," *Journal of Neuroscience* 39 (2019): 6035–37.

23. Antonio Russo et al., "Pathophysiology of Migraine: What Have We Learned from Functional Imaging?" *Current Neurology and Neuroscience Reports* 17 (2017): 95–107.

24. Soo-Jin Cho et al., "Fibromyalgia among Patients with Chronic Migraine and Chronic Tension-Type Headache: A Multicenter Prospective Cross-Sectional Study," *Headache* 58 (2018): 311–13.

25. Farnaz Amoozegar, "Depression Comorbidity in Migraine," *International Review of Psychiatry* 29 (2017): 504–15.

26. Marcelo Bigal et al., "Prevalence and Characteristics of Allodynia in Headache Sufferers," *Neurology* 70 (2008): 1525–33.

27. Beard, *Practical Treatise on Nervous Exhaustion*.

28. Headache Classification Subcommittee of the International Headache Society (IHS), *The International Classification of Headache Disorders*, 2nd ed., in *Cephalalgia: An International Journal of Headache* 24, Suppl. 1 (2004): 1–160.

29. Mervyn J. Eadie, "Ergot of Rye: The First Specific for Migraine," *Journal of Clinical Neuroscience* 11 (2004): 4–7.

30. Michael Anthony and James W. Lance, "The Role of Serotonin in Migraine," in *Modern Topics in Migraine*, ed. J. Pearce (London: Heinemann Medical, 1975), 107–23.

31. Roger K. Cady et al., "Treatment of Acute Migraine with Subcutaneous Sumatriptan," *Journal of the American Medical Association* 265 (1991): 2831–35.

32. Jakob Møller Hansen et al., "Calcitonin Gene-Related Peptide Triggers Migraine-Like Attacks in Patients with Migraine with Aura," *Cephalalgia: An International Journal of Headache* 30 (2010): 1179–86.

33. Katrin Probyn et al., "Prognostic Factors for Chronic Headache: A Systematic Review," *Neurology* 89 (2017): 291–301.

34. Francis Graham Crookshank, *Migraine and Other Common Neuroses* (London: Kegan Paul, Trench, Trubner & Co., 1926; London: Routledge, 2016). Citations refer to the Routledge edition.

7. TENSION HEADACHES; JAW AND FACIAL PAIN

1. Rigmor H. Jensen, "Tension-Type Headache: The Normal and Most Prevalent Headache," *Headache* 58 (2018): 339–45.

2. Robert M. Bennett and Don L. Goldenberg, "Fibromyalgia, Myofascial Pain, Tender Points and Trigger Points: Splitting or Lumping?" *Arthritis Research and Therapy* 30 (2011): 117–20.

3. Lasse-Marius Honningsvag et al., "White Matter Hyperintensities and Headache: A Population-Based Study (HUNT MRI)," *Cephalalgia* 38 (2018): 1927–39.

4. Line Buchgreitz et al., "Frequency of Headache Is Related to Sensitization: A Population Study," *Pain* 123 (2006): 19–27.

5. Marcela Romero-Reyes and James M. Uyanik, "Orofacial Pain Management: Current Perspectives," *Journal of Pain Research* 7 (2014): 99–115.

6. Eric Schiffman et al., "Diagnostic Criteria for Temporomandibular Disorders (DC/TMD) for Clinical and Research Applications: Recommendations of the International RDC/TMD Consortium Network and Orofacial Pain Special Interest Group," *Journal of Oral Facial Pain Headache* 28 (2014): 6–27.

7. Ibid.

8. Ibid.

9. Zorina-Lichtenwalter et al., "Genetic Predictors of Human Chronic Pain Conditions."

10. Chia-shu Lin, "Brain Signature of Chronic Orofacial Pain: A Systematic Review and Meta-Analysis on Neuroimaging Research of Trigeminal Neuropathic Pain and Temporomandibular Joint Disorders," *PLoS One* 9, no. 4 (2014): e94300. doi:10.1371/journal.pone.0094300.

11. Imen Ayouni et al., "Comorbidity between Fibromyalgia and Temporomandibular Disorders: A Systematic Review," *Oral Surgery, Oral Medicine, Oral Pathology, Oral Radiology* 128, no. 1 (2019): 33–42.

12. Vegard Strøm et al., *Effect of Surgical Treatment for Temporomandibular Disorders* (Oslo: Norwegian Knowledge Centre for the Health Services, 2013).

13. Romero-Reyes and Uyanik, "Orofacial Pain Management."

14. Bennett and Goldenberg, "Fibromyalgia, Myofascial Pain, Tender Points and Trigger Points."

15. Mohammed S. Alrashdan and Mustafa Alkhader, "Psychological Factors in Oral Mucosa and Orofacial Pain Conditions," *European Journal of Dentistry* 11 (2017): 548–52.

8. CHRONIC LOW BACK AND NECK PAIN; THE ROLE OF TRAUMA AND INJURY

1. Hayden Herrera, *Frida: A Biography of Frida Kahlo* (New York: Harper & Row, 1983), 507.

2. Carol A. Courtney, Michael A. O'Hearn, and Carla C. Franck, "Frida Kahlo: Portrait of Chronic Pain," *Physical Therapy* 97 (2017): 90–96.

3. Ibid.

4. Manuel Martinez-Lavin et al., "Fibromyalgia in Frida Kahlo's Life and Art," *Arthritis Rheumatology* 43 (2000): 708–9.

5. Richard A. Deyo and James N. Weinstein, "Low Back Pain," *New England Journal of Medicine* 344 (2001): 363–70.

6. Institute of Medicine, *Relieving Pain in America*.

7. Deyo and Weinstein, "Low Back Pain."

8. Maureen C. Jensen et al., "Magnetic Resonance Imaging of the Lumbar Spine in People without Back Pain," *New England Journal of Medicine* 331 (1994): 69–73.

9. Ibid.

10. Ibid.

11. Kliment Gatzinsky et al., "Optimizing the Management and Outcomes of Failed Back Surgery Syndrome: A Proposal of a Standardized Multidisciplinary Team Care Pathway," *Pain Research Management*, July 8, 2019. doi:10.1155/2019/8184592.

12. Allen Lebovits et al., "Struck from Behind: Maintaining Quality of Life with Chronic Low Back Pain," *Journal of Pain* 10 (2009): 927–31.

13. Douglas Gross et al., "A Population-Based Survey of Back Pain Beliefs in Canada," *Spine* 31 (2006): 2142–45.

14. Deyo and Weinstein, "Low Back Pain."

15. Lena Nordeman, Ronny Gunnarsson, and Kaisa Mannerkorpi, "Prevalence and Characteristics of Widespread Pain in Female Primary

Health Care Patients with Chronic Low Back Pain," *Clinical Journal of Pain* 28 (2012): 65–72.

16. Jeroen Kregel et al., "Structural and Functional Brain Abnormalities in Chronic Low Back Pain: A Systematic Review," *Seminars in Arthritis and Rheumatism* 45 (2015): 229–37.

17. Kara J. Bragg and Matthew Varacallo, "Cervical (Whiplash) Sprain," in *Stat*Pearls (Treasure Island, FL: StatPearls Publishing, 2019), https://www.ncbi.nlm.nih.gov/books/NBK541016.

18. Robert Ferrari, Anthony S. Russell, Linda J. Carroll, and J. David Cassidy, "A Re-Examination of the Whiplash Associated Disorders (WAD) as a Systemic Illness," *Annals of Rheumatic Diseases* 64 (2005): 1337–42.

19. Barbara Cagnie et al., "Is Traumatic and Non-Traumatic Neck Pain Associated with Brain Alterations? A Systematic Review," *Pain Physician* 20 (2017): 245–60.

20. Pooria Sarrami et al., "Factors Predicting Outcome in Whiplash Injury: A Systematic Meta-Review of Prognostic Factors," *Journal of Orthopaedic Traumatology* 18 (2017): 9–16.

21. Eric Rydman et al., "Long-Term Follow-Up of Whiplash Injuries Reported to Insurance Companies: A Cohort Study on Patient-Reported Outcomes and Impact of Financial Compensation," *European Spine Journal* 27 (2018): 1255–61.

22. Mark Awerbuch, "Repetitive Strain Injuries: Has the Australian Epidemic Burnt Out?" *Internal Medicine Journal* 34 (2004): 416–19.

23. Ibid.

24. Geoff O. Littlejohn, "Key Issues in Repetitive Strain Injury," in *Fibromyalgia, Chronic Fatigue Syndrome and Repetitive Strain Injury*, ed. A. Chalmers et al. (New York: Hayworth Medical Press, 1995), 25–33.

25. Denise Grady, "In One Country, Chronic Whiplash Is Uncompensated (and Unknown)," *New York Times*, May 7, 1996.

26. Ibid.

9. COMPLEX REGIONAL PAIN AND NEUROPATHIC PAIN

1. Kevin B. Guthmiller and Matthew Varacallo, "Complex Regional Pain Syndrome (CRPS), Reflex Sympathetic Dystrophy (RSD)," in *Stat-*

Pearls (Treasure Island, FL: StatPearls Publishing, 2019), https://www.ncbi.nlm.nih.gov/books/NBK430719.

2. Ibid.

3. Katherine Dutton and Geoffrey Littlejohn, "Terminology, Criteria, and Definitions in Complex Regional Pain Syndrome: Challenges and Solutions," *Journal of Pain Research* 8 (2015): 871–77.

4. Ibid.

5. Ibid.

6. En Lin Goh, Swathikan Chidambaram, and Daqing Ma, "Complex Regional Pain Syndrome: A Recent Update," *Burns & Trauma* 5 (2017): 2. doi:10.1186/s41038-016-0066-4.

7. Pallai Shillo et al., "Painful and Painless Diabetic Neuropathies: What Is the Difference?" *Current Diabetes Reports* 19 (2019): 32, https://doi.org/10.1007/s11892-019-1150-5.

8. Ibid.

9. Dylan Henssen et al., "Alterations in Grey Matter Density and Functional Connectivity in Trigeminal Neuropathic Pain and Trigeminal Neuralgia: A Systematic Review and Meta-Analysis," *Neuroimage: Clinical* 24 (2019): 102039, https://doi.org/10.1016/j.nicl.2019.102039.

10. Steven P. Cohen, "Neuropathic Pain: Mechanisms and Their Clinical Implications," *British Medical Journal* 348 (2014): f7656.

11. Lindsay Zilliox, "Neuropathic Pain: Selected Topics in Outpatient Neurology," *CONTINUUM: Lifelong Learning in Neurology* 23, no. 2 (2017): 512–32. doi:10.1212/CON.0000000000000462.

12. H. Shim et al., "Complex Regional Pain Syndrome: A Narrative Review for the Practicing Clinician," *British Journal of Anaesthesia* 2 (2019): e424–33.

13. Melanie Racine, "Chronic Pain and Suicide Risk: A Comprehensive Review," *Progress in Neuro-Psychopharmacology and Biological Psychiatry* 87 (2018): 269–80.

14. Amy S. B. Bohnert and Mark A. Ilgen, "Understanding Links among Opioid Use, Overdose, and Suicide," *New England Journal of Medicine* 380, no 1. (January 2019): 71–79.

10. CHRONIC BOWEL, BLADDER, AND PELVIC PAIN

1. Alexander C. Ford, Brian E. Lacy, and Nicholas J. Talley, "Irritable Bowel Syndrome," *New England Journal of Medicine* 376 (2017): 2566–78.

2. Daniel J. Clauw, "Fibromyalgia and Related Conditions," *Mayo Clinic Proceedings* 90 (2015): 680–92.

3. Michiko Kano et al., "Understanding Neurogastroenterology from Neuroimaging Perspective: A Comprehensive Review of Functional and Structural Brain Imaging in Functional Gastrointestinal Disorders," *Journal of Gastroenterology and Motility* 24, no. 4 (2018): 512–27.

4. Elisabet Johannesson et al., "Physical Activity Improves Symptoms in Irritable Bowel Syndrome: A Randomized Controlled Trial," *American Journal of Gastroenterology* 106, no. 5 (2011): 915–22.

5. J. Quentin Clemens et al., "The MAPP Research Network: A Novel Study of Urologic Chronic Pelvic Pain Syndromes," *BMC Urology* 14 (2014): 57. doi:10.1186/1471-2490-14-57.

6. Ibid.

7. Steven Harte et al., "Quantitative Assessment of Non-Pelvic Pressure Pain Sensitivity in Urologic Chronic Pelvic Pain Syndrome: A MAPP Research Network Study," *Pain* 160 (2019): 1270–80.

8. Ibid.

9. Niloofar Afari et al., "A MAPP Network Case-Control Study of Urologic Chronic Pelvic Pain Compared with Non-Urologic Pain Conditions," *Clinical Journal of Pain* 36, no. 1 (2020): 8–15. doi:10.1097/AJP.0000000000000769.

10. Davis C. Woodworth et al., "Changes in Brain White Matter Structure Are Associated with Urine Proteins in Urologic Chronic Pelvic Pain Syndrome (UCPPS): A MAPP Network Study," *PLos One* 13, no. 12 (December 5, 2018): e0206807. doi:10.1371/journal.pone.0206807.

11. Michael E. Hyland et al., "Symptom Frequency and Development of a Generic Functional Disorder Symptom Scale Suitable for Use in Studies of Patients with Irritable Bowel Syndrome, Fibromyalgia Syndrome or Chronic Fatigue Syndrome," *Chronic Diseases and Translational Medicine* 5 (2019): 129–38.

12. John W. Warren, Patricia Langenberg, and Daniel J. Clauw, "The Number of Existing Functional Somatic Syndromes (FSSs) Is an Impor-

tant Risk Factor for New, Different FSSs," *Journal of Psychosomatic Research* 74, no. 1 (2013): 12–17.

13. Hyland et al., "Symptom Frequency and Development of a Generic Functional Disorder Symptom Scale."

11. ARTHRITIS AND CHRONIC PAIN

1. Ernest Vina and C. Kwoh, "Epidemiology of Osteoarthritis: Literature Update," *Current Opinion in Rheumatology* 30 (2018): 160–67.

2. Ibid.

3. Ibid.

4. Ibid.

5. Nicholas D. Clement and David J. Deehan, "Overweight and Obese Patients Require Total Hip and Total Knee Arthroplasty at a Younger Age," *Journal of Orthopedic Research* (September 3, 2019). doi:10.1002/jor.24460.

6. Ibid.

7. Marc C. Hochberg et al., "American College of Rheumatology 2012 Recommendations for the Use of Nonpharmacologic and Pharmacologic Therapies in Osteoarthritis of the Hand, Hip, and Knee," *Arthritis Care Research* 64, no. 4 (2012): 465–74.

8. Lucía Gato-Calvo et al., "Platelet-Rich Plasma in Osteoarthritis Treatment: Review of Current Evidence," *Therapeutic Advances in Chronic Disease* 10, no. 4 (February 2019). doi:10.1177/2040622319825567.

9. Marc C. Hochberg et al., "Combined Chondroitin Sulfate and Glucosamine for Painful Knee Osteoarthritis: A Multicentre, Randomised, Double-Blind, Non-Inferiority Trial versus Celecoxib," *Annals of Rheumatic Diseases* 75, no. 1 (January 2016): 37–44. doi:10.1136/annrheumdis-2014-206792.

10. Thomas J. Schnitzer et al., "Effect of Tanezumab on Joint Pain, Physical Function, and Patient Global Assessment of Osteoarthritis among Patients with Osteoarthritis of the Hip or Knee: A Randomized Clinical Trial," *Journal of the American Medical Association* 322 (2019): 37–48.

11. Patrick H. Finan et al., "Discordance between Pain and Radiographic Severity in Knee Osteoarthritis: Findings from Quantitative Sen-

sory Testing of Central Sensitization," *Arthritis Rheumatology* 65, no. 2 (2013): 363–72.

12. Ibid.

13. Stephen E. Gwilym et al., "Thalamic Atrophy Associated with Painful Osteoarthritis of the Hip Is Reversible after Arthroplasty: A Longitudinal Voxel-Based Morphometric Study," *Arthritis Rheumatology* 62, no. 10 (2010): 293040.

14. Ibid.

15. Gwyn N. Lewis et al., "Structural Brain Alterations before and after Total Knee Arthroplasty: A Longitudinal Assessment," *Pain Medicine* 19 (2018): 2166–76.

16. Xia Liao et al., "Brain Gray Matter Alterations in Chinese Patients with Chronic Knee Osteoarthritis Pain Based on Voxel-Based Morphometry," *Medicine* (Baltimore) 97, no. 12 (March 2018): e0145.

17. David T. Felson et al., "Multiple Nonspecific Sites of Joint Pain outside the Knees Develop in Persons with Knee Pain," *Arthritis Rheumatology* 69 (2017): 335–42.

18. Alan M. Rathbun et al., "Dynamic Effects of Depressive Symptoms on Osteoarthritis Knee Pain," *Arthritis Care & Research* 70 (2018): 80–88.

19. Bindee Kuriya et al., "High Disease Activity Is Associated with Self-Reported Depression and Predicts Persistent Depression in Early Rheumatoid Arthritis," *Journal of Rheumatology* 45 (2018): 1101–108.

20. Sizheng Steven Zhao, Stephen J. Duffield, and Nicola J. Goodson, "The Prevalence and Impact of Comorbid Fibromyalgia in Inflammatory Arthritis," *Best Practice & Research Clinical Rheumatology* 33, no. 3 (June 2019): 101423. doi:10.1016/j.berh.2019.06.005.

21. Ibid.

22. Marco L. Loggia and Robert R. Edwards, "Brain Structural Alterations in Chronic Knee Osteoarthritis: What Can Treatment Effects Teach Us?" *Pain Medicine* 19 (2018): 2099–2100.

23. Chad M. Brummett et al., "Characteristics of Fibromyalgia Independently Predict Poorer Long-Term Analgesic Outcomes Following Total Knee and Hip Arthroplasty," *Arthritis Rheumatology* 67 (2015): 1386–94.

12. PHARMACOLOGIC THERAPY

1. Diarmuid Jeffreys, *Aspirin: The Remarkable Story of a Wonder Drug* (New York: Bloomsbury, 2008).

2. Kok Yuen Ho et al., "Nonsteroidal Anti-Inflammatory Drugs in Chronic Pain: Implications of New Data for Clinical Practice," *Journal of Pain Research* 11 (2018): 1937–48.

3. Don L. Goldenberg, "Pharmacological Treatment of Fibromyalgia and Other Chronic Musculoskeletal Pain," *Best Practice and Research in Clinical Rheumatology* 21 (2007): 499–511.

4. Ibid.

5. Ibid.

6. Chao Zeng et al., "Association of Tramadol with All-Cause Mortality among Patients with Osteoarthritis," *Journal of the American Medical Association* 321 (2019): 969–82.

7. Olivier Bruyere et al., "An Updated Algorithm Recommendation for the Management of Knee Osteoarthritis from the European Society for Clinical and Economic Aspects of Osteoporosis, Osteoarthritis and Musculoskeletal Diseases (ESCEO)," *Seminars in Arthritis and Rheumatism*, April 30, 2019. doi:10.1016/j.semarthrit.2019.04.00.

13. THE OPIOID CRISIS; CANNABIS

1. Elisabeth Astyrakaki, Alexandra Papaioannou, and Helen Askitopoulou, "References to Anesthesia, Pain, and Analgesia in the Hippocratic Collection," *Anesthesia & Analgesia* 110 (2010): 188–94.

2. Michael J. Brownstein, "A Brief History of Opiates, Opioid Peptides, and Opioid Receptors," *Proceedings of the National Academy of Sciences of the United States of America* 90 (1993): 5391–92.

3. Ibid.

4. Josh Sanborn, "Heroin Is Being Laced with a Terrifying New Substance: What to Know about Carfentanil," *Time*, September 12, 2016.

5. Ibid.

6. Roger Chou et al., "Research Gaps on Use of Opioids for Chronic Noncancer Pain: Findings from a Review of the Evidence for an

American Pain Society and American Academy of Pain Medicine Clinical Practice Guideline," *Journal of Pain* 10 (2009): 147–59.

7. Ibid.

8. Nora D. Volkow and A. Thomas McLellan, "Opioid Abuse in Chronic Pain: Misconceptions and Mitigation Strategies," *New England Journal of Medicine* 374 (2016): 1253–63.

9. Ibid.

10. Ibid.

11. Art Van Zee, "The Promotion and Marketing of OxyContin: Commercial Triumph, Public Health Tragedy," *American Journal of Public Health* 99 (2009): 221–27.

12. Ibid.

13. Ibid.

14. Jason W. Busse et al., "Opioids for Chronic Noncancer Pain: A Systematic Review and Meta-Analysis," *Journal of the American Medical Association* 320 (2018): 2448–60.

15. Don L. Goldenberg et al., "Opioid Use in Fibromyalgia: A Cautionary Tale," *Mayo Clinic Proceedings* 91 (2016): 640–48.

16. Sonja Vučković et al., "Cannabinoids and Pain: New Insights from Old Molecules," *Frontiers in Pharmacology* 9 (November 13, 2018): 1259. doi:10.3389/fphar.2018.01259.

17. Ivan Urits et al., "An Update of Current Cannabis-Based Pharmaceuticals in Pain Medicine," *Pain Therapy* 8 (2019): 41–51.

18. Ibid.

19. Mary Ann Fitzcharles and Winfred Häuser, "Cannabinoids in the Management of Musculoskeletal or Rheumatic Diseases," *Current Rheumatology Report* 18 (2016): 76–82.

20. Martin Mucke et al., "Cannabis-Based Medicines for Chronic Neuropathic Pain in Adults," *Cochrane Database of Systematic Reviews*, March 7, 2018. doi:10.1002/14651858.CD012182.

21. Madeline H. Meiera et al., "Persistent Cannabis Users Show Neuropsychological Decline from Childhood to Midlife," *Proceedings of the National Academy of Sciences of the United States of America* 109 (2012): E2657–64.

22. Kevin F. Boehnke et al., "High-Frequency Medical Cannabis Use Is Associated with Worse Pain among Individuals with Chronic Pain," *Journal of Pain*, September 24, 2019. doi:10.1016/j.jpain.2019.09.006.

23. Austin Frakt, "Can Marijuana Help Cure the Opioid Crisis?" *New York Times*, June 17, 2019.

24. Ibid.

14. EXERCISE

1. Rodrigo Da Silva Santos and Giovane Galdino, "Endogenous Systems Involved in Exercise-Induced Analgesia," *Journal of Physiology and Pharmacology* 69 (2018): 3–13.

2. Ibid.

3. Matthew Jones et al., "Aerobic Training Increases Pain Tolerance in Healthy Individuals," *Medicine & Science in Sports & Exercise* 46 (2014): 1640–47.

4. Laura D. Ellingson et al., "Exercise Strengthens Central Nervous System Modulation of Pain in Fibromyalgia," *Brain Sciences* 6, no. 1 (February 26, 2016).

5. Ibid.

6. Elizabeth L. Whitlock et al., "Association between Persistent Pain and Memory Decline and Dementia in a Longitudinal Cohort of Elders," *Journal of the American Medical Association Internal Medicine* 177 (2017): 1146–53.

7. Eduardo Fontes et al., "Modulation of Cortical and Subcortical Brain Areas at Low and High Exercise Intensities," *British Journal of Sports Medicine* (August 16, 2019). doi:10.1136/bjsports-2018-100295.

8. Joseph Firth et al., "Effect of Aerobic Exercise on Hippocampal Volume in Humans: A Systematic Review and Meta-Analysis," *Neuroimage* 166 (2018): 230–38; Peter A. Hall et al., "Neuroimaging, Neuromodulation, and Population Health: The Neuroscience of Chronic Disease Prevention," *Annals of the New York Academy of Sciences* 1428 (2018): 240–56.

9. Tina D. Hoang et al., "Effect of Early Adult Patterns of Physical Activity and Television Viewing on Midlife Cognitive Function," *Journal of the American Medical Association Psychiatry* 73 (2016): 73–79.

10. Julia Bidonde et al., "Aerobic Exercise Training for Adults with Fibromyalgia," *Cochrane Database of Systematic Reviews* 6, no. 6 (June 21, 2017): CD012700. doi:10.1002/14651858.CD012700.

11. Blanca Gavilan-Carrera et al., "Substituting Sedentary Time with Physical Activity in Fibromyalgia and the Association with Quality of Life and Impact of the Disease: The Al-Ándalus Project," *Arthritis Care and Res earch* 71 (2019): 281–89.

12. Xian-Guo Meng and Shou-Wei Yue, "Efficacy of Aerobic Exercise for Treatment of Chronic Low Back Pain: A Meta-Analysis," *American Journal of Physical Medicine & Rehabilitation* 94 (2015): 358–65.

13. Faisal Mohammed Amin et al., "The Association between Migraine and Physical Exercise," *Journal of Headache and Pain* 19 (2018): 83–90.

14. Małgorzata Eliks, Małgorzata Zgorzalewicz-Stachowiak, and Krystyna Zeńczak-Praga, "Application of Pilates-Based Exercises in the Treatment of Chronic Non-Specific Low Back Pain: State of the Art," *Postgraduate Medical Journal* 95 (2019): 41–45.

15. Grace H. Lo et al., "Evidence That Swimming May Be Protective of Knee Osteoarthritis: Data from the Osteoarthritis Initiative," *Physical Medicine & Rehabilitation*, October 19, 2019. doi:10.1002/pmrj.12267.

16. Grace H. Lo et al., "Running Does Not Increase Symptoms or Structural Progression in People with Knee Osteoarthritis: Data from the Osteoarthritis Initiative," *Clinical Rheumatology* 37 (2018): 2497–504.

17. Ibid.

18. Huan-Ji Dong et al., "Is Excess Weight a Burden for Older Adults Who Suffer Chronic Pain?" *Bio Medical Central Geriatrics* 18 (2018): 270–80.

19. Elizabeth G. VanDenKerkhof et al., "Diet, Lifestyle and Chronic Widespread Pain: Results from the 1958 British Birth Cohort Study," *Pain Research and Management* 16 (2011): 87–92.

20. Dmitry Tumin et al., "Weight Gain Trajectory and Pain Interference in Young Adulthood: Evidence from a Longitudinal Birth Cohort Study," *Pain Medicine*, August 6, 2019. doi:10.1093/pm/pnz184.

21. Akiko Okifuji and Bradford D. Hare, "The Association between Chronic Pain and Obesity," *Journal of Pain Research* 8 (2015): 399–408.

22. Ibid.

23. Andrew Schrepf et al., "Improvement in the Spatial Distribution of Pain, Somatic Symptoms, and Depression after a Weight Loss Intervention," *Journal of Pain* 18 (2017): 1542–50.

24. Damon L. Swift et al., "The Role of Exercise and Physical Activity in Weight Loss and Maintenance," *Progress in Cardiovascular Diseases* 56 (2014): 441–47.

25. Dennis T. Villareal et al., "Aerobic or Resistance Exercise, or Both, in Dieting Obese Older Adults," *New England Journal of Medicine* 376 (2017): 1943–55.

26. Cameron W. Foreman et al., "Total Joint Arthroplasty in the Morbidly Obese," *Journal of Arthroplasty*, August 17, 2019. doi:10.1016/j. arth.2019.08.019.

27. Bryan D. Springer et al., "What Are the Implications of Withholding Total Joint Arthroplasty in the Morbidly Obese?" *Bone and Joint Journal* 101-B, no. 7_Supple_C (July 2019): 28–32. doi:10.1302/0301-620X.101B7.BJJ-2018-1465.R1.

28. Ibid.

29. Alexander S. McLawhorn et al., "Bariatric Surgery Improves Outcomes after Lower Extremity Arthroplasty in the Morbidly Obese," *Journal of Arthroplasty* 33 (2018): 2062–69.

15. COMPLEMENTARY AND ALTERNATIVE MEDICINE, INCLUDING YOGA, TAI CHI, AND ACUPUNCTURE

1. Tainya C. Clarke et al., "Trends in the Use of Complementary Health Approaches among Adults: United States, 2002–2012," *National Health Statistics Reports* 79 (2015): 1–16.

2. Ibid.

3. Ibid.

4. Ibid.

5. Richard L. Nahin, Barbara J. Stussman, and Patricia M. Herman, "Out of Pocket Expenditures on Complementary Health Approaches Associated with Painful Health Conditions in a Nationally Representative Adult Sample," *Journal of Pain* 15 (2015): 362–72.

6. Claudia Wang et al., "Trends in Yoga, Tai Chi, and Qigong Use among US Adults, 2002–2017," *American Journal of Public Health* 109 (2019): 755–61.

7. Yin Wu et al., "Yoga as Antihypertensive Lifestyle Therapy: A Systematic Review and Meta-Analysis," *Mayo Clinic Proceedings* 94 (2019): 432–46.

8. Chenchen Wang et al., "A Randomized Trial of Tai Chi for Fibromyalgia," *New England Journal of Medicine* 363 (2010): 743–54.

9. Chenchen Wang et al., "Effect of Tai Chi versus Aerobic Exercise for Fibromyalgia: Comparative Effectiveness Randomized Controlled Trial," *British Medical Journal* 360 (2018): k851. doi:10.1136/bmj.k851.

10. Angus Yu et al., "Revealing the Neural Mechanisms Underlying the Beneficial Effects of Tai Chi: A Neuroimaging Perspective," *American Journal of Chinese Medicine* 46 (2018): 231–59.

11. Roger Chou et al., "Nonpharmacologic Therapies for Low Back Pain: A Systematic Review for an American College of Physicians Clinical Practice Guideline," *Annals of Internal Medicine* 166 (2017): 493–505.

12. Kathryn Curtis et al., "An Eight-Week Yoga Intervention Is Associated with Improvements in Pain, Psychological Functioning and Mindfulness, and Changes in Cortisol Levels in Women with Fibromyalgia," *Journal of Pain Research* 4 (2011): 189–201.

13. Rahul Saxena et al., "Effects of Yogic Intervention on Pain Scores and Quality of Life in Females with Chronic Pelvic Pain," *International Journal of Yoga* 10 (2017): 9–15.

14. James W. Carson et al., "Mindful Yoga Pilot Study Shows Modulation of Abnormal Pain Processing in Fibromyalgia Patients," *International Journal of Yoga Therapy* 26 (2016): 93–100.

15. Richard L. Nahin et al., "Evidence-Based Evaluation of Complementary Health Approaches for Pain Management in the United States," *Mayo Clinic Proceedings* 91 (2016): 1292–306.

16. Zhang Xin-chang et al., "Acupuncture Therapy for Fibromyalgia: A Systematic Review and Meta-Analysis of Randomized Controlled Trials," *Journal of Pain Research* 12 (2019): 527–42.

17. Rupali P. Dhond et al., "Neuroimaging Acupuncture Effects in the Human Brain," *Journal of Alternative and Complementary Medicine* 13 (2007): 603–16.

18. Ather Ali et al., "Massage Therapy and Quality of Life in Osteoarthritis of the Knee: A Qualitative Study," *Pain Medicine* 18 (2017): 1168–75.

19. Nahin et al., "Evidence-Based Evaluation of Complementary Health Approaches."

20. Ibid.

21. Ana Rita Silva et al., "Dietary Interventions in Fibromyalgia: A Systematic Review," *Annals of Medicine* 51, suppl. (2019): 2–14. doi:10.1080/07853890.2018.1564360.

22. Sarah E. E. Miles, Karen P. Nicholson, and Blair H. Smith, "Chronic Pain: A Review of Its Epidemiology and Associated Factors in Population-Based Studies," *British Journal of Anaesthesia* 123 (2019): e273–83.

23. Kimball C. Atwood IV, "Naturopathy, Pseudoscience, and Medicine: Myths and Fallacies vs. Truth," *Medscape General Medicine* 6, no. 1 (2004): 33.

24. Ibid.

25. Silva et al., "Dietary Interventions in Fibromyalgia."

26. Atwood, "Naturopathy, Pseudoscience, and Medicine."

16. MIND-BODY THERAPY

1. Jon Kabat-Zinn, *Full Catastrophe Living* (New York: Random House, 1990).

2. Ken H. Kaplan, Don L. Goldenberg, and Maureen Galvin-Nadeau, "The Impact of a Meditation-Based Stress Reduction Program on Fibromyalgia," *General Hospital Psychiatry* 15 (1993): 284–89.

3. Adrienne L. Adler-Neal and Fedal Zeidan, "Mindfulness Meditation for Fibromyalgia: Mechanistic and Clinical Considerations," *Current Rheumatology Reports* 19 (2017): 59.

4. José G. Luiggi-Hernandez et al., "Mindfulness for Chronic Low Back Pain: A Qualitative Analysis," *Pain Medicine* 19 (2018): 2138–45.

5. Adler-Neal and Zeidan, "Mindfulness Meditation for Fibromyalgia."

6. Ivan Urits et al., "An Update on Cognitive Therapy for the Management of Chronic Pain: A Comprehensive Review," *Current Pain and Headache Report* 10 (2019): 57.

7. Marta Alda et al., "Effectiveness of Cognitive Behaviour Therapy for the Treatment of Catastrophisation in Patients with Fibromyalgia: A Randomised Controlled Trial," *Arthritis Research &Therapy* 13 (2011): R173.

8. Mark Lumley et al., "Emotional Awareness and Expression Therapy, Cognitive Behavioral Therapy, and Education for Fibromyalgia: A Cluster-Randomized Controlled Trial," *Pain* 158 (2017): 2354–63.

9. Christina McCrae et al., "Gray Matter Changes Following Cognitive Behavioral Therapy for Patients with Comorbid Fibromyalgia and Insomnia: A Pilot Study," *Journal of Clinical and Sleep Medicine* 14 (2018): 1595–603; David A. Seminowicz et al., "Cognitive-Behavioral Therapy Increases Prefrontal Cortex Gray Matter in Patients with Chronic Pain," *Journal of Pain* 14 (2013): 1573–84.

10. Adler-Neal and Zeidan, "Mindfulness Meditation for Fibromyalgia."

11. Swati Mehta, Vanessa A. Peynenburg, and Heather D. Hadjistavropoulos, "Internet-Delivered Cognitive Behaviour Therapy for Chronic Health Conditions: A Systematic Review and Meta-Analysis," *Journal of Behavioral Medicine* 42 (2019): 169–87.

12. Robert Sielski, Winfred Rief, and Julia Anna Glombiewski, "Efficacy of Biofeedback in Chronic Low Back Pain: A Meta-Analysis," *International Journal of Behavioral Medicine* 24 (2017): 25–41.

13. Jamie L. Rhudy et al., "Modified Biofeedback (Conditioned Biofeedback) Promotes Anti-Nociception by Increasing the Nociceptive Flexion Reflex Threshold and Reducing Temporal Summation of Pain: A Controlled Trial," *Journal of Pain*, November 1, 2019. doi:10.1016/j.jpain.2019.10.006.

14. Antonio Del Casale et al., "Pain Perception and Hypnosis: Findings from Recent Functional Neuroimaging Studies," *International Journal of Clinical and Experimental Hypnosis* 63 (2015): 144–70.

15. Chelsea M. Cummiford et al., "Changes in Resting State Functional Connectivity after Repetitive Transcranial Direct Current Stimulation Applied to Motor Cortex in Fibromyalgia Patients," *Arthritis Research & Therapy* 18 (2016): 40.

16. Aline P. Brietzke et al., "Large Treatment Effect with Extended Home-Based Transcranial Direct Current Stimulation over Dorsolateral Prefrontal Cortex in Fibromyalgia: A Proof of Concept Sham-Randomized Clinical Study," *Journal of Pain*, July 26, 2019. doi:10.1016/j.jpain.2019.06.013.

17. Carol G. T. Vance et al., "Development of a Method to Maximize the Transcutaneous Electrical Nerve Stimulation Intensity in Women with Fibromyalgia," *Journal of Pain Research* 11 (2018): 2269–78.

17. FINDING THE RIGHT
HEALTH-CARE TEAM

1. Institute of Medicine, *Relieving Pain in America.*
2. Ibid.
3. Deepak Doltani et al., "Who Accompanies Patients to the Chronic Pain Clinic?" *Irish Journal of Medical Science* 186 (2017): 235–38.
4. John W. Burns et al., "Spouse and Patient Beliefs and Perceptions about Chronic Pain: Effects on Couple Interactions and Patient Pain Behavior," *Journal of Pain*, April 5, 2019. doi:10.1016/j.jpain.2019.04.001.
5. Luz Canovas et al., "Impact of Empathy in the Patient-Doctor Relationship on Chronic Pain Relief and Quality of Life," *Pain Medicine* 19 (2018): 1304–14.
6. Maxie Blasini et al., "The Role of Patient-Practitioner Relationships in Placebo and Nocebo Phenomena," *International Review in Neurobiology* 138 (2018): 211–31.
7. Ibid.; Lindsey C. McKernan et al., "Outpatient Engagement and Predicted Risk of Suicide Attempts in Fibromyalgia," *Arthritis Care & Research* 71 (2019): 1255–63.

18. YOUR PERSONAL GUIDE TO MANAGING CHRONIC PAIN

1. Lewis Thomas, *The Medusa and the Snail* (New York: Viking Press, 1979).
2. Institute of Medicine, *Relieving Pain in America.*
3. Chad M. Brummett et al., "Characteristics of Fibromyalgia Independently Predict Poorer Long-Term Analgesic Outcomes Following Total Knee and Hip Arthroplasty," *Arthritis Rheumatology* 67 (2015): 1386–94.
4. Marianne S. Matthias and Matthew J. Bair, "The Patient–Provider Relationship in Chronic Pain Management: Where Do We Go from Here?" *Pain Medicine* 11 (2010): 1747–49.
5. Ibid.
6. Ibid.

7. T. M. Damush et al., "Pain Self-Management Training Increases Self-Efficacy, Self-Management Behaviours and Pain and Depression Outcomes," *European Journal of Pain* 20, no. 7 (2016): 1070–78. doi:10.1002/ejp.830.

8. Kurt Kroenke et al., "Telecare Collaborative Management of Chronic Pain in Primary Care: A Randomized Clinical Trial," *Journal of the American Medical Association* 312 (2014): 240–48.

9. Susan Reisine et al., "Employment and Health Status Changes among Women with Fibromyalgia: A Five-Year Study," *Arthritis and Rheumatology* 59 (2008): 1735–41.

10. Institute of Medicine, *Relieving Pain in America.*

11. Ibid.

12. Elaine Scarry, *The Body in Pain: The Making and Unmaking of the World* (New York: Oxford University Press, 1985).

BIBLIOGRAPHY

Abbey, Susan E., and Paul E Garfinkel. "Neurasthenia and Chronic Fatigue Syndrome: The Role of Culture in the Making of a Diagnosis." *American Journal of Psychiatry* 148 (1991): 1638–46.

Adler-Neal, Adrienne L., and Fedal Zeidan. "Mindfulness Meditation for Fibromyalgia: Mechanistic and Clinical Considerations." *Current Rheumatology Reports* 19 (2017). 59.

Afari, Niloofar, Dedra Buchwald, Daniel Clauw, Barry Hong, Xiaoling Hou, John Krieger, Chris Mullins, Alisa J. Stephens-Shields, Marianna Gasperi, and David A. Williams. "A MAPP Network Case-Control Study of Urologic Chronic Pelvic Pain Compared with Non-Urologic Pain Conditions." *Clinical Journal of Pain* 36, no.1 (2020): 8–15. doi:10.1097/AJP.0000000000000769.

Alda, Marta, Juan V. Luciano, Eva Andrés, Antoni Serrano-Blanco, Baltasar Rodero, Yolanda López del Hoyo, Miquel Roca, Sergio Moreno, Rosa Magallón, and Javier Garcia-Campayo. "Effectiveness of Cognitive Behaviour Therapy for the Treatment of Catastrophisation in Patients with Fibromyalgia: A Randomised Controlled Trial." *Arthritis Research & Therapy* 13 (2011): R173.

Ali, Ather, Lisa Rosenberger, Theresa Weiss, Carl Milak, and Adam I. Perlman. "Massage Therapy and Quality of Life in Osteoarthritis of the Knee: A Qualitative Study." *Pain Medicine* 18 (2017): 1168–75.

Alrashdan, Mohammed S., and Mustafa Alkhader. "Psychological Factors in Oral Mucosa and Orofacial Pain Conditions." *European Journal of Dentistry* 11 (2017): 548–52.

Alvarez, Walter. "The Migrainous Personality and Constitution." *American Journal of the Medical Sciences* 213 (1947): 1–8.

American Geriatrics Society Panel on Pharmacological Management of Persistent Pain in Older Persons. "Pharmacologic Management of Persistent Pain in Older Persons." *Journal of the American Geriatric Society* 57 (2009): 1331–39.

Amin, Faisal Mohammed, Stavroula Aristeidou, Carlo Baraldi, Ewa K. Czapinska-Ciepiela, Daponte D. Ariadni, Davide Di Lenola, Cherilyn Fenech, Konstantinos Kampouris, Giorgos Karagiorgis, Mark Braschinsky et al. "The Association between Migraine and Physical Exercise." *Journal of Headache and Pain* 19 (2018): 83–90.

Amoozegar, Farnaz. "Depression Comorbidity in Migraine." *International Review of Psychiatry* 29 (2017): 504–15.

Andersen, Hans Christian. *The Princess and the Pea*. Copenhagen: C. A. Reitzel, 1835.

Andoh, Jamila, Martin Diers, Christopher Milde, Christopher Frobel, and Herta Flor. "Neural Correlates of Evoked Phantom Limb Sensations." *Biological Psychology* 126 (2017): 89–97.

Anthony, Michael, and James W. Lance. "The Role of Serotonin in Migraine." In *Modern Topics in Migraine*, edited by J. Pearce, 107–23. London: Heinemann Medical, 1975.

Arnold, Lesley M., James I. Hudson, Evelyn V. Hess, Avis E. Ware, Deborah A. Fritz, Megan B. Auchenbach, Linsey O. Starck, and Paul E. Keck. "Family Study of Fibromyalgia." *Arthritis Rheumatology* 50 (2004): 944–52.

Aroke, Edwin A., Paula V. Joseph, Abhrarup Roy, Demario S. Overstreet, Trygve O. Tollefsbol, David E. Vance, and Burel R. Goodin. "Could Epigenetics Help Explain Racial Disparities in Chronic Pain?" *Journal of Pain Research* 12 (2019): 701–10.

Astyrakaki, Elisabeth, Alexandra Papaioannou, and Helen Askitopoulou. "References to Anesthesia, Pain, and Analgesia in the Hippocratic Collection." *Anesthesia & Analgesia* 110 (2010): 188–94.

Atwood, Kimball C., IV. "Naturopathy, Pseudoscience, and Medicine: Myths and Fallacies vs. Truth." *Medscape General Medicine* 6, no. 1 (2004): 33.

Awerbuch, Mark. "Repetitive Strain Injuries: Has the Australian Epidemic Burnt Out?" *Internal Medicine Journal* 34 (2004): 416–19.

Ayouni, Imen, Raja Chebbi, Zeglaoui Hela, and Monia Dhidah. "Comorbidity between Fibromyalgia and Temporomandibular Disorders: A Systematic Review." *Oral Surgery, Oral Medicine, Oral Pathology, Oral Radiology* 128, no. 1 (2019): 33–42.

Bair, Matthew J., Rebecca L Robinson, Wayne Katon, and Kurt Kroenke. "Depression and Pain Comorbidity: A Literature Review." *Archives of Internal Medicine* 163 (2003): 2433–45.

Beard, George. *A Practical Treatise on Nervous Exhaustion*. New York: W. Wood, 1880.

Benigeri, Mike, and Pierre Pluye. "Shortcomings of Health Information on the Internet." *Health Promotion International* 18 (2003): 381–86.

Bennett, Robert M., and Don L. Goldenberg. "Fibromyalgia, Myofascial Pain, Tender Points and Trigger Points: Splitting or Lumping?" *Arthritis Research and Therapy* 30 (2011): 117–20.

Bidonde, Julia, Angela J. Busch, Candice L. Schachter, Tom J. Overend, Soo Y. Kim, Suelen M. Goes, Catherine Boden, and Heather J. A. Foulds. "Aerobic Exercise Training for Adults with Fibromyalgia." *Cochrane Database of Systematic Reviews* 6, no. 6 (June 21, 2017): CD012700. doi:10.1002/14651858.CD012700.

Bigal, Marcelo, Sait Ashina, R. Burstein, Michael L. Reed, Dawn Buse, Daniel Serrano, and Richard B. Lipton. "Prevalence and Characteristics of Allodynia in Headache Sufferers." *Neurology* 70 (2008): 1525–33.

Blanchard, Melvin, Hector D. Molina-Vicenty, Phyllis K. Stein, Xue Li, Joel Karlinsky, Renee Alpern, Domenic J. Reda, and Rosemary Toomey. "Medical Correlates of Chronic Multisymptom Illness in Gulf War Veterans." *American Journal of Medicine* 132 (2019): 510–18.

Blasini, Maxie, Nathalie Peiris, Thelma Wright, and Luana Colloca. "The Role of Patient-Practitioner Relationships in Placebo and Nocebo Phenomena." *International Review in Neurobiology* 138 (2018): 211–31.

Boehnke, Kevin F., J. Ryan Scott, Evangelos Litinas, Suzanne Sisley, David A. Williams, and Daniel J. Clauw. "High-Frequency Medical Cannabis Use Is Associated with Worse Pain among Individuals with Chronic Pain." *Journal of Pain*, September 24, 2019. doi:10.1016/j.jpain.2019.09.006.

Bohnert, Amy S. B., and Mark A. Ilgen. "Understanding Links among Opioid Use, Overdose, and Suicide." *New England Journal of Medicine* 380, no. 1 (January 2019): 71–79.

Bragg, Kara J., and Matthew Varacallo. "Cervical (Whiplash) Sprain." In *StatPearls*. Treasure Island, FL: StatPearls Publishing, 2019. https://www.ncbi.nlm.nih.gov/books/NBK541016.

Brietzke, Aline P., Maxciel Zortea, Fabiana Carvalho, Paulo R. S. Sanches, Danton P. Silva Jr., Iraci Lucena da Silva Torres, Felipe Fregni, and Wolnei Caumo. "Large Treatment Effect with Extended Home-Based Transcranial Direct Current Stimulation over Dorsolateral Prefrontal Cortex in Fibromyalgia: A Proof of Concept Sham-Randomized Clinical Study." *Journal of Pain*, July 26, 2019. doi:10.1016/j.jpain.2019.06.013.

Brownstein, Michael J. "A Brief History of Opiates, Opioid Peptides, and Opioid Receptors." *Proceedings of the National Academy of Sciences of the United States of America* 90 (1993): 5391–92.

Brummett, Chad M., Andrew G. Urquhart, Afton L. Hassett, Alex Tsodikov, Brian R. Hallstrom, Nathan I. Wood, David Alan Williams, and Daniel J. Clauw. "Characteristics of Fibromyalgia Independently Predict Poorer Long-Term Analgesic Outcomes Following Total Knee and Hip Arthroplasty." *Arthritis Rheumatology* 67 (2015): 1386–94.

Bruyere, Olivier, Germain Honvo, Nicola Veronese, Nigel K. Arden, Jaime Branco, Elizabeth M. Curtis, Nasser M. Al-Daghri, Gabriel Herrero-Beaumont, Johanne Martel-Pelletier, and Jean-Pierre Pelletier. "An Updated Algorithm Recommendation for the Management of Knee Osteoarthritis from the European Society for Clinical and Economic Aspects of Osteoporosis, Osteoarthritis and Musculoskeletal Diseases (ESCEO)." *Seminars in Arthritis and Rheumatism*, April 30, 2019. doi:10.1016/j.semarthrit.2019.04.00.

Buchgreitz, Line, A. Lyngnerg, Lars Bendtsen, and Rigmor Jensen. "Frequency of Headache Is Related to Sensitization: A Population Study." *Pain* 123 (2006): 19–27.

Burns, John W., Kristina M. Post, David A. Smith, Laura S. Porter, Asokumar Buvanendran, Anne Marie Fras, and Francis J. Keefe. "Spouse and Patient Beliefs and Perceptions about Chronic Pain: Effects on Couple Interactions and Patient Pain Behavior." *Journal of Pain*, April 5 2019. doi:10.1016/j.jpain.2019.04.001.

Busse, Jason W., Li Wang, Mostafa Kamaleldin, Samantha Craigie, John J. Riva, Luis Montoya, Sohail M. Mulla, Luciane Lopes, Nicole Vogel, Eric Chen et al. "Opioids for Chronic Noncancer Pain: A Systematic Review and Meta-Analysis." *Journal of the American Medical Association* 320 (2018): 2448–60.

Butler, Laura, and Nadine Foster. "Back Pain Online: A Cross-Sectional Survey of the Quality of Web-Based Information on Low Back Pain." *Spine* 28 (2003): 395–401.

Cady, Roger K., Jeanette K. Wendt, John R. Kirchner, Joseph D. Sargent, John F. Rothrock, and Harold Skaggs. "Treatment of Acute Migraine with Subcutaneous Sumatriptan." *Journal of the American Medical Association* 265 (1991): 2831–35.

Cagnie, Barbara, Lieven Danneels, Karen Caeyenberghs, Mira Meeus, Iris Coppieters, and Robby DePauw. "Is Traumatic and Non-Traumatic Neck Pain Associated with Brain Alterations? A Systematic Review." *Pain Physician* 20 (2017): 245–60.

Canovas, Luz, Antonio-José Carrascosa, Modesto García, Mariano Fernandez, Vicente Monsalve, and José-Francisco Soriano. "Impact of Empathy in the Patient-

Doctor Relationship on Chronic Pain Relief and Quality of Life." *Pain Medicine* 19 (2018): 1304–14.

Carrington, Charles. *Rudyard Kipling: His Life and Work*. London: Macmillan, 1955.

Carson, James W., Kimberly M. Carson, Kim D. Jones, Lindsay Lancaster, and Scott D. Mist. "Mindful Yoga Pilot Study Shows Modulation of Abnormal Pain Processing in Fibromyalgia Patients." *International Journal of Yoga Therapy* 26 (2016): 93–100.

Chen, Longtu, Sheikh J. Ilham, and Bin Feng. "Pharmacological Approach for Managing Pain in Irritable Bowel Syndrome." *Anesthesiology and Pain Medicine* 7 (2017): e42747.

Cho, Soo-Jin, Jong-Hee Sohn, Jong Seok Bae, and Min Kyung Chu. "Fibromyalgia among Patients with Chronic Migraine and Chronic Tension-Type Headache: A Multicenter Prospective Cross-Sectional Study." *Headache* 58 (2018): 311–13.

Chou, Roger, Jane C. Ballantyne, Gilbert J. Fanciullo, Perry G. Fine, and Christine Miaskowski. "Research Gaps on Use of Opioids for Chronic Noncancer Pain: Findings from a Review of the Evidence for an American Pain Society and American Academy of Pain Medicine Clinical Practice Guideline." *Journal of Pain* 10 (2009): 147–59.

Chou, Roger, Richard Deyo, Janna Friedly, Andrea Skelly, Robin Hashimoto, Melissa Weimer, Rongwei Fu, Tracy L. Dana, Paul Kraegel, and Jessica Griffin. "Nonpharmacologic Therapies for Low Back Pain: A Systematic Review for an American College of Physicians Clinical Practice Guideline." *Annals of Internal Medicine* 166 (2017): 493–505.

Clarke, Tainya C., Lindsey I. Black, Barbara J. Stussman, Patricia M. Barnes, and Richard L. Nahin. "Trends in the Use of Complementary Health Approaches among Adults: United States, 2002–2012." *National Health Statistics Reports* 79 (2015): 1–16.

Clauw, Daniel J. "Fibromyalgia and Related Conditions." *Mayo Clinic Proceedings* 90 (2015): 680–92.

Clemens, J. Quentin, Chris Mullins, John W. Kusek, Ziya Kirkali, Emeran A. Mayer, Larissa V. Rodríguez, David J. Klumpp, Anthony J. Schaeffer, Karl J. Kreder, Dedra Buchwald et al. "The MAPP Research Network: A Novel Study of Urologic Chronic Pelvic Pain Syndromes." *BMC Urology* 14 (2014): 57. doi:10.1186/1471-2490-14-57.

Clement, Nicholas D., and David J. Deehan. "Overweight and Obese Patients Require Total Hip and Total Knee Arthroplasty at a Younger Age." *Journal of Orthopedic Research* (September 3, 2019). doi:10.1002/jor.24460.

Cline, R. J. W, and K. M. Haynes. "Consumer Health Information Seeking on the Internet: The State of the Art." *Health Education Research* 16 (2001): 671–92.

Coffelt, Thomas A., Benjamin D. Bauer, and Aaron E. Carroll. "Inpatient Characteristics of the Child Admitted with Chronic Pain." *Pediatrics* 132, no. 2 (2013): e422.

Cohen, Steven P. "Neuropathic Pain: Mechanisms and Their Clinical Implications." *British Medical Journal* 348 (2014): f7656.

Coiro, Pierluca, and Daniela D. Pollak. "Sex and Gender Bias in the Experimental Neurosciences." *Translational Psychiatry* 9 (2019): 90–98.

Collins, Kassondra L., Hannah G. Russell, Patrick J. Schumacher, Katherine E. Robinson-Freeman, Ellen C. O'Conor, Kyla D. Gibney et al. "A Review of Current Theories and Treatments for Phantom Limb Pain." *Journal of Clinical Investigation* 128 (2018): 2168–76.

Courtney, Carol A., Michael A. O'Hearn, and Carla C. Franck. "Frida Kahlo: Portrait of Chronic Pain." *Physical Therapy* 97 (2017): 90–96.

Cox, James J., Frank Reimann, Adeline K. Nicholas, Gemma Thornton, Emma Roberts, Kelly Springell, Guishan Karbani, Hussain Jafri, Jovaria Mannan, Yasmin Raashid et al. "An SCN9A Channelopathy Causes Congenital Inability to Experience Pain." *Nature* 444 (2006): 894–98.

Crookshank, Francis Graham. *Migraine and Other Common Neuroses*. London: Kegan Paul, Trench, Trubner & Co., 1926. Reprinted. London: Routledge, 2016. References are to the 2016 edition.

Cummiford, Chelsea M., Thiago Nascimento, Bradley R. Foerster, Daniel J. Clauw, Jon-Kar Zubieta, Richard E. Harris, and Alexandre F. DaSilva. "Changes in Resting State Functional Connectivity after Repetitive Transcranial Direct Current Stimulation Applied to Motor Cortex in Fibromyalgia Patients." *Arthritis Research & Therapy* 18 (2016): 40.

Curtis, Kathryn, Anna Osadchuk, and Joel Katz. "An Eight-Week Yoga Intervention Is Associated with Improvements in Pain, Psychological Functioning and Mindfulness, and Changes in Cortisol Levels in Women with Fibromyalgia." *Journal of Pain Research* 4 (2011): 189–201.

D'Aoust, Rita F., Alicia Gill Rossiter, Amanda Elliott, Ming Ji, Cecile Lengacher, and Maureen Groer. "Women Veterans, a Population at Risk for Fibromyalgia: The Associations between Fibromyalgia, Symptoms, and Quality of Life." *Military Medicine* 182, no. 7 (2017): e1828–35.

Da Silva Santos, R., and Giovane Galdino. "Endogenous Systems Involved in Exercise-Induced Analgesia." *Journal of Physiology and Pharmacology* 69 (2018): 3–13.

Dahlhamer, James, Jacqueline Lucas, Richard Nahin, Sean Mackey, Lynn DeBar, Robert Kerns, Michael Von Korff, Linda Porter, and Charles Helmick. "Prevalence of Chronic Pain and High-Impact Chronic Pain among Adults: United States, 2016." *Morbidity and Mortality Weekly Report* 67, no. 36 (September 14, 2018): 1001–6. doi:10.15585/mmwr.mm6736a2.

Damien, Janie Luana Colloca, Carmen-Édith Bellei-Rodriguez, and Serge Marchand. "Pain Modulation: From Conditioned Pain Modulation to Placebo and Nocebo Effects in Experimental and Clinical Pain." *International Review of Neurobiology* 139 (2018): 255–96.

Damush, T. M., K. Kroenke, M. J. Bair, J. Wu, W. Tu, E. E. Krebs, and E. Poleshuck. "Pain Self-Management Training Increases Self-Efficacy, Self-Management Behaviours and Pain and Depression Outcomes." *European Journal of Pain* 20, no. 7 (2016): 1070–78. doi:10.1002/ejp.830.

Daniel, Britt Talley. *Migraine*. Bloomington, IN: AuthorHouse, 2010.

Daraz, Lubna, Joy C. MacDermid, Seanne Wilkins, Jane Gibson, and Lynn Shaw. "The Quality of Websites Addressing Fibromyalgia: An Assessment of Quality and Readability Using Standardised Tools." *British Medical Journal Open* 1, no. 1 (2011): e000152.

Del Casale, Antonio, Stefano Ferracuti, Chiara Rapinesi, Daniele Serata, Saverio Simone Caltagirone, Valeria Savoja, Daria Piacentino, Gemma Callovini, Giovanni Manfredi, and Gabriele Sani. "Pain Perception and Hypnosis: Findings from Recent Functional Neuroimaging Studies." *International Journal of Clinical and Experimental Hypnosis* 63 (2015): 144–70.

Deyo, Richard A., and James N. Weinstein. "Low Back Pain." *New England Journal of Medicine* 344 (2001): 363–70.

Dhond, Rupali P., Norman Kettner, and Vitaly Napadow. "Neuroimaging Acupuncture Effects in the Human Brain." *Journal of Alternative and Complementary Medicine* 13 (2007): 603–16.

Doltani, Deepak, Ather Imran, Jean Saunders, and Dominic Harmon. "Who Accompanies Patients to the Chronic Pain Clinic?" *Irish Journal of Medical Science* 186 (2017): 235–38.

Dong, Huan-Ji, Britt Larsson, Lars-Åke Levin, Lars Bernfort, and Björn Gerdle. "Is Excess Weight a Burden for Older Adults Who Suffer Chronic Pain ?" *Bio Medical Central Geriatrics* 18 (2018): 270–80.

Donohue, Julie M., Marisa Cevasco, and Meredith B. Rosenthal. "A Decade of Direct-to-Consumer Advertising of Prescription Drugs." *New England Journal of Medicine* 357 (2007): 673–81.

Dorado, Kathleen, Kristin L. Schreiber, Alexandra Koulouris, Robert R. Edwards, Vitaly Napadow, and Asimina Lazaridou. "Interactive Effects of Pain Catastrophizing and Mindfulness on Pain Intensity in Women with Fibromyalgia." *Health Psychology Open* 5, no. 2 (October 22, 2018). doi:10.1177/2055102918807406.

Dumit, Joseph. "Pharmaceutical Witnessing: Drugs for Life in an Era of Direct-to-Consumer Advertising." In *The Pharmaceutical Studies Reader*, edited by Sergio Sismondo and Jeremy A. Greene, 33–47. Manchester, UK: Wiley Blackwell, 2015.

Dutton, Katherine, and Geoffrey Littlejohn. "Terminology, Criteria, and Definitions in Complex Regional Pain Syndrome: Challenges and Solutions." *Journal of Pain Research* 8 (2015): 871–77.

Eadie, Mervyn J. "Ergot of Rye: The First Specific for Migraine." *Journal of Clinical Neuroscience* 11 (2004): 4–7.

Eliks, Małgorzata, Małgorzata Zgorzalewicz-Stachowiak, and Krystyna Zeńczak-Praga. "Application of Pilates-Based Exercises in the Treatment of Chronic Non-Specific Low Back Pain: State of the Art." *Postgraduate Medical Journal* 95 (2019): 41–45.

Ellingson, Laura D., Aaron J. Stegner, Isaac J. Schwabacher, Kelli F. Koltyn, and Dane B. Cook. "Exercise Strengthens Central Nervous System Modulation of Pain in Fibromyalgia." *Brain Sciences* 6, no. 1 (February 26, 2016).

Eysenbach, Gunther, John Powell, and Oliver Kuss. "Empirical Studies Assessing the Quality of Health Information for Consumers on the World Wide Web: A Systematic Review." *Journal of the American Medical Association* 287 (2002): 2691–700.

Felson, David T., Jingbo Niu, Emily A. Quinn, Tuhina Neogi, Cara Lewis, Cora E. Lewis, Laura A. Frey Law, Chuck McCulloch, Michael Nevitt, and Michael P. Lavalley. "Multiple Nonspecific Sites of Joint Pain outside the Knees Develop in Persons with Knee Pain." *Arthritis Rheumatology* 69 (2017): 335–42.

Ferrari, Robert, Anthony S. Russell, Linda J. Carroll, and J. David Cassidy. "A Re-Examination of the Whiplash Associated Disorders (WAD) as a Systemic Illness." *Annals of Rheumatic Diseases* 64 (2005): 1337–42.

Finan, Patrick H., Luis F. Buenaver, Sara C. Bounds, Shahid Hussain, Raymond J. Park, Uzma J. Haque, Claudia Campbell, Jennifer A. Haythornthwaite, Robert R. Edwards, and M. T. Smith. "Discordance between Pain and Radiographic Severity in Knee Osteoarthritis: Findings from Quantitative Sensory Testing of Central Sensitization." *Arthritis Rheumatology* 65, no. 2 (2013): 363–72.

Firth, Joseph, Brendon Stubbs, Davy Vancampfort, Felipe Schuch, Jim Lagopoulos, Simon Rosenbaum, and Philip B. Ward. "Effect of Aerobic Exercise on Hippocampal Volume in Humans: A Systematic Review and Meta-Analysis." *Neuroimage* 166 (2018): 230–38.

Fitzcharles, Mary Ann, and Winfred Häuser. "Cannabinoids in the Management of Musculoskeletal or Rheumatic Diseases." *Current Rheumatology Report* 18 (2016): 76–82.

Fontes, Eduardo, Henrique Bortolotti, Kell Grandjean da Costa, Brunno Machado de Campos, Gabriela K. Castanho, Rodrigo Hohl, Timothy Noakes, and Li Li Min. "Modulation of Cortical and Subcortical Brain Areas at Low and High Exercise Intensities." *British Journal of Sports Medicine*, August 16, 2019. doi:10.1136/bjsports-2018-100295.

Ford, Alexander C., Brian E. Lacy, and Nicholas J. Talley. "Irritable Bowel Syndrome." *New England Journal of Medicine* 376 (2017): 2566–78.

Foreman, Cameron W., John J. Callaghan, Timothy S. Brown, Jacob M. Elkins, and Jesse E. Otero. "Total Joint Arthroplasty in the Morbidly Obese." *Journal of Arthroplasty*, August 17, 2019. doi:10.1016/j.arth.2019.08.019.

Freburger, Janet K., George M. Holmes, Robert P. Agans, Anne M. Jackman, Jane D. Darter, Andrea S. Wallace, Liana D. Castel, William D. Kalsbeek, and Timothy S. Carey. "The Rising Prevalence of Chronic Low Back Pain." *Archives Internal Medicine* 169 (2009): 251–58.

Fuchs, Xaver, Herta Flor, and Robin Bekrater-Bodmann. "Psychological Factors Associated with Phantom Limb Pain: A Review of Recent Findings." *Pain Research Management* 2018, no. 5080123 (June 21, 2018). doi:10.1155/2018/5080123.

Gato-Calvo, Lucía, Joana Magalhaes, Cristina Ruiz-Romero, Francisco J. Blanco, and Elena F. Burguera. "Platelet-Rich Plasma in Osteoarthritis Treatment: Review of Current Evidence." *Therapeutic Advances in Chronic Disease* 10, no. 4 (February 2019). doi:10.1177/2040622319825567.

Gatzinsky, Kliment, Sam Eldabe, Jean-Philippe Deneuville, Wim Duyvendak, Nicolas Naiditch, Jean-Pierre Van Buyten, and Philippe Rigoard. "Optimizing the Management and Outcomes of Failed Back Surgery Syndrome: A Proposal of a Standardized Multidisciplinary Team Care Pathway." *Pain Research Management* July 8, 2019. doi:10.1155/2019/8184592.

Gavilan-Carrera, Blanca, Victor Segura-Jimenez, Rania A. Mekary, Milkana Borges-Cosic, Pedro Acosta Manzano, Fer Estevez-Lopez, Immaculada Alvarez-Gallardo, Rinie Geenen, and Manuel Delgado-Fernandez. "Substituting Sedentary Time with Physical Activity in Fibromyalgia and the Association with Quality of Life and Impact of the Disease: The Al-Ándalus Project." *Arthritis Care and Research* 71 (2019): 281–89.

Gendelman, Omer, Howard Amital, Yael Bar-On, Dana Ben-Ami Shor, Daniela Amital, Shmuel Tiosano, Varda Shalev, and Gabriel Chodick. "Time to Diagnosis of Fibromyalgia and Factors Associated with Delayed Diagnosis in Primary Care." *Best Practice & Research Clinical Rheumatology* 32 (2018): 489–99.

Gereau, Robert W., IV, Kathleen A. Sluka, William Maixner, Seddon R. Savage, Theodore J. Price, Beth B. Murinson, Mark D. Sullivan, and Roger B. Fillingim. "A Pain Research Agenda for the 21st Century." *Journal of Pain* 15 (2014): 1203–14.

Gerring, Zachary F., Allan F. McRae, Grant W. Montgomery, and Dale R. Nyholt. "Genome-Wide DNA Methylation Profiling in Whole Blood Reveals Epigenetic Signatures Associated with Migraine." *BMC Genomics* 19 (2018): 69–79.

Goh, En Lin, Swathikan Chidambaram, and Daqing Ma. "Complex Regional Pain Syndrome: A Recent Update." *Burns & Trauma* 5 (2017): 2. doi:10.1186/s41038-016-0066-4.

Goldenberg, Don L. "Fibromyalgia Syndrome a Decade Later: What Have We Learned?" *Archives of Internal Medicine* 159 (1999): 777–85.

Goldenberg, Don L. "Fibromyalgia: To Diagnose or Not. Is That Still the Question?" *Journal of Rheumatology* 31, no. 4 (May 2004): 633–35.

Goldenberg, Don L. "Fibromyalgia: Why Such Controversy?" *Annals of Rheumatic Diseases* 54 (1995): 3–5.

Goldenberg, Don L. "Pharmacological Treatment of Fibromyalgia and Other Chronic Musculoskeletal Pain." *Best Practice and Research in Clinical Rheumatology* 21 (2007): 499–511.

Goldenberg, Don L., Daniel J. Clauw, Robert E. Palmer, and Andrew G. Clair. "Opioid Use in Fibromyalgia: A Cautionary Tale." *Mayo Clinic Proceedings* 91 (2016): 640–48.

Goldenberg, Don L., and Hartej S. Sandhu. "Fibromyalgia and Post-Traumatic Stress Disorder." *Seminars in Arthritis and Rheumatism* 32 (2002): 1–2.

Gormley, Padhraig, Bendik S. Winsvold, Dale R. Nyholt, Mikko Kallela, Daniel I. Chasman, and Aarno Palotie. "Migraine Genetics: From Genome-Wide Association Studies to Translational Insights." *Genome Medicine* 8 (2016): 86. doi:10.1186/s13073-016-0346-4.

Gowers, William R. *The Border-Land of Epilepsy*. London: Churchill, 1907.

Grady, Denise. "In One Country, Chronic Whiplash Is Uncompensated (and Unknown)." *New York Times*, May 7, 1996.

Gross, Douglas, Robert Ferrari, Anthony Russell, Michele Battié, Donald Schopflocher, Richard Hu, Gordon Waddell, and Rachelle Buchbinder. "A Population-Based Survey of Back Pain Beliefs in Canada." *Spine* 31 (2006): 2142–45.

Guthmiller, Kevin B., and Matthew Varacallo. "Complex Regional Pain Syndrome (CRPS), Reflex Sympathetic Dystrophy (RSD)." In *StatPearls*. Treasure Island, FL: StatPearls Publishing, 2019. https://www.ncbi.nlm.nih.gov/books/NBK430719.

Gwilym, Stephen E., Nicola Filippini, Gwenaelle Douaud, Andrew J. Carr, and Irene Tracey. "Thalamic Atrophy Associated with Painful Osteoarthritis of the Hip Is Reversible after Arthroplasty: A Longitudinal Voxel-Based Morphometric Study." *Arthritis Rheumatology* 62, no. 10 (2010): 293040.

Habib, Abdella M., Andrei L. Okorokov, Matthew N. Hill, Jose T. Bras, Man-Cheung Lee, Shengnan Li, Samuel J. Gossage, Marie van Drimmelen, Maria Morena, Henry Houlden et al. "Microdeletion in a FAAH Pseudogene Identified in a Patient with High Anandamide Concentrations and Pain Insensitivity." *British Journal of Anaesthesia* 123 (2019): 249–53.

Hall, Peter A., Warren K. Bickel, Kirk I. Erickson, and Dylan D. Wagner. "Neuroimaging, Neuromodulation, and Population Health: The Neuroscience of Chronic Disease Prevention." *Annals of the New York Academy of Sciences* 1428 (2018): 240–56.

Hansen, Jakob Møller, Anne Werner Hauge, Jes Olesen, and Messoud Ashina. "Calcitonin Gene-Related Peptide Triggers Migraine-Like Attacks in Patients with Migraine with Aura." *Cephalalgia: An International Journal of Headache* 30 (2010): 1179–86.

Harte, Steven, Andrew Schrepf, Robert Gallop, Grant Kruger, Hing Hung Lai, Siobhan Sutcliffe, Megan Halvorson, Eric Ichesco, Bruce D. Naliboff, Niloofar Afari et al. "Quantitative Assessment of Non-Pelvic Pressure Pain Sensitivity in Urologic Chronic Pelvic Pain Syndrome: A MAPP Research Network Study." *Pain* 160 (2019): 1270–80.

Häuser, Winfried, Alexandra Galek, Brigitte Erbslöh-Möller, Volker Köllner, Hedi Kühn-Becker, Jost Langhorst, Franz Petermann, Ulrich Prothmann, Andreas Winkelmann, Gabriele Schmutzer et al. "Posttraumatic Stress Disorder in Fibromyalgia Syndrome: Prevalence, Temporal Relationship between Posttraumatic Stress and Fibromyalgia Symptoms, and Impact on Clinical Outcome." *Pain* 154 (2013): 1216–23.

Haygarth, John. *Of the Imagination, as a Cause and as a Cure of Disorders of the Body, Exemplified by Fictitious Tractors, and Epidemical Convulsions*. Bath, England: Crutwell, 1801.

Headache Classification Subcommittee of the International Headache Society (IHS). *The International Classification of Headache Disorders*. 2nd ed. In *Cephalalgia: An International Journal of Headache* 24, Suppl. 1 (2004): 1–160.

Heckert, Justin. "The Hazards of Growing Up Painlessly." *New York Times*, November 15, 2012.

Henssen, Dylan, Jurriaan Dijk, Robin Knepfle, Matthijs Sieffers, Anouk Winter, and Kris Vissers. "Alterations in Grey Matter Density and Functional Connectivity in Trigeminal Neuropathic Pain and Trigeminal Neuralgia: A Systematic Review and

Meta-Analysis." *Neuroimage: Clinical* 24 (2019): 102039. https://doi.org/10.1016/j.nicl.2019.102039.

Herrera, Hayden. *Frida: A Biography of Frida Kahlo.* New York: Harper & Row, 1983.

Hirsh, Adam, Nicole Hollingshead, Matthew Bair, Marianne Matthias, and Kurt Kroenke. "Preferences, Experience, and Attitudes in the Management of Chronic Pain and Depression: A Comparison of Physicians and Medical Students." *Clinical Journal of Pain* 30 (2014): 766–84.

Ho, Kok Yuen, Kok Ann Gwee, Yew Kuang Cheng, Kam Hon Yoon, Hwan Tak Hee, and Abdul Razakjr Omar. "Nonsteroidal Anti-Inflammatory Drugs in Chronic Pain: Implications of New Data for Clinical Practice." *Journal of Pain Research* 11 (2018): 1937–48.

Hoang, Tina D., Jared Reis, Na Zhu, David R. Jacobs Jr., Lenore J. Launer, Rachel A. Whitmer, Stephen Sidney, and Kristine Yaffe. "Effect of Early Adult Patterns of Physical Activity and Television Viewing on Midlife Cognitive Function." *Journal of the American Medical Association Psychiatry* 73 (2016): 73–79.

Hochberg, Marc C., Roy D. Altman, Karine Toupin April, Maria Benkhalti, Gordon Guyatt, Jessie Mcgowan, Tanveer Towheed, Vivian Welch, George Wells, and Peter Tugwell. "American College of Rheumatology 2012 Recommendations for the Use of Nonpharmacologic and Pharmacologic Therapies in Osteoarthritis of the Hand, Hip, and Knee." *Arthritis Care Research* 64, no. 4 (2012): 465–74.

Hochberg, Marc C., Johanne Martel-Pelletier, Jordi Monfort, Ingrid Möller, Juan Ramón Castillo, Nigel Arden, Francis Berenbaum, Francisco J. Blanco, Philip G. Conaghan, Gema Doménech et al. "Combined Chondroitin Sulfate and Glucosamine for Painful Knee Osteoarthritis: A Multicentre, Randomised, Double-Blind, Non-Inferiority Trial versus Celecoxib." *Annals of Rheumatic Diseases* 75, no. 1 (January 2016): 37–44. doi:10.1136/annrheumdis-2014-206792.

Honningsvag, Lasse-Marius, Asta Kristine Haberg, Knut Hagen, Kjell Arne Kvistad, Lars Jacob Stovner, and Mattias Linde. "White Matter Hyperintensities and Headache: A Population-Based Study (HUNT MRI)." *Cephalalgia* 38 (2018): 1927–39.

Hyland, Michael E., Allison M. Bacon, Joseph W. Lanario, and Anthony F. Davies. "Symptom Frequency and Development of a Generic Functional Disorder Symptom Scale Suitable for Use in Studies of Patients with Irritable Bowel Syndrome, Fibromyalgia Syndrome or Chronic Fatigue Syndrome." *Chronic Diseases and Translational Medicine* 5 (2019): 129–38.

Institute of Medicine Committee on Advancing Pain Research, Care, and Education. *Relieving Pain in America: A Blueprint for Transforming Prevention, Care, Education, and Research.* Washington, DC: National Academies Press, 2011.

Jeffreys, Diarmuid. *Aspirin: The Remarkable Story of a Wonder Drug.* New York: Bloomsbury, 2008.

Jensen, Maureen C., Michael N. Brant-Zawadzki, Nancy Obuchowski, Michael T. Modic, Dennis Malkasian, and Jeffrey S. Ross. "Magnetic Resonance Imaging of the Lumbar Spine in People without Back Pain." *New England Journal of Medicine* 331 (1994): 69–73.

Jensen, Rigmor H. "Tension-Type Headache: The Normal and Most Prevalent Headache." *Headache* 58 (2018): 339–45.

Ji, Ru-Rong, Andrea Nackley, Yul Huh, Niccolo Terrando, and William Maixner. "Neuroinflammation and Central Sensitization in Chronic and Widespread Pain." *Anesthesiology* 129 (2018): 343–66.

Johannesson, Elisabet, Magnus Simrén, Hans Strid, Antal Bajor, and Riadh Sadik. "Physical Activity Improves Symptoms in Irritable Bowel Syndrome: A Randomized Controlled Trial." *American Journal of Gastroenterology* 106, no. 5 (2011): 915–22.

Jones, Gareth T., Barbara I. Nicholl, John McBeth, Kelly A. Davies, Richard K. Morriss, Chris Dickens, and Gary J. Macfarlane. "Role of Road Traffic Accidents and Other Traumatic Events in the Onset of Chronic Widespread Pain: Results from a Population-Based Prospective Study." *Arthritis Care & Research* 63 (2011): 696–701.

Jones, Matthew, John Booth, Janet Taylor, and Benjamin Barry. "Aerobic Training Increases Pain Tolerance in Healthy Individuals." *Medicine & Science in Sports & Exercise* 46 (2014): 1640–47.

Kabat-Zinn, Jon. *Full Catastrophe Living*. New York: Random House, 1990.

Kano, Michiko, Patrick Dupont, Qasim Aziz, and Shin Fukudo. "Understanding Neurogastroenterology from Neuroimaging Perspective: A Comprehensive Review of Functional and Structural Brain Imaging in Functional Gastrointestinal Disorders." *Journal of Gastroenterology and Motility* 24, no. 4 (2018): 512–27.

Kaplan, Ken H., Don L. Goldenberg, and Maureen Galvin-Nadeau. "The Impact of a Meditation-Based Stress Reduction Program on Fibromyalgia." *General Hospital Psychiatry* 15 (1993): 284–89.

Kerr, Jasmine I., and Andrea Burri. "Genetic and Epigenetic Epidemiology of Chronic Widespread Pain." *Journal of Pain Research* 10 (2017): 2021–29.

Krause, Adam J., Aric A. Prather, Tor D. Wager, Martin A. Lindquist, and Matthew P. Walker. "The Pain of Sleep Loss: A Brain Characterization in Humans." *Journal of Neuroscience* 39 (2019): 2291–300.

Kregel, Jeroen, Mira Meeus, Anneleen Malfliet, Mieke Dolphens, Lieven Danneels, and Barbara Cagnie. "Structural and Functional Brain Abnormalities in Chronic Low Back Pain: A Systematic Review." *Seminars in Arthritis and Rheumatism* 45 (2015): 229–37.

Kroenke, Kurt, Erin E. Krebs, Jingwei Wu, Zhangsheng Yu, Neale R. Chumbler, and Matthew Bair. "Telecare Collaborative Management of Chronic Pain in Primary Care: A Randomized Clinical Trial." *Journal of the American Medical Association* 312 (2014): 240–48.

Kuriya, Bindee, Raman Joshi, Mohammad Movahedi, Emmanouil Rampakakis, John S. Sampalis, Claire Bombardier, and Ontario Best Practices Research Initiative Investigators. "High Disease Activity Is Associated with Self-Reported Depression and Predicts Persistent Depression in Early Rheumatoid Arthritis." *Journal of Rheumatology* 45 (2018): 1101–108.

Larach, Daniel B., Michael J. Sahara, Sawsan As-Sanie, Stephanie Moser, Andrew G. Urquhart, Jules Lin, Joseph A. Wakeford, Daniel J. Clauw, Jennifer F. Waljee, and Chad M. Brummett. "Patient Factors Associated with Opioid Consumption in the Month Following Major Surgery." *Annals of Surgery*, August 5, 2019. doi:10.1097/SLA.0000000000003509.

Lebovits, Allen, Brian Hainline, Laura S. Stone, David A. Seminowicz, James T. Brunz, Richard W. Rosenquist, and Penney Cowan. "Struck from Behind: Maintaining Quality of Life with Chronic Low Back Pain." *Journal of Pain* 10 (2009): 927–31.

Lee, UnCheol, Minkyung Kim, Kyoungeun Lee, Chelsea M. Kaplan, Daniel J. Clauw, Seunghwan Kim, George A. Mashour, and Richard E. Harris. "Functional Brain Network Mechanism of Hypersensitivity in Chronic Pain." *Scientific Reports* 8 (2018): 243–66.

Lewis, Gwyn N., Rosalind S. Parker, Sheena Sharma, David A. Rice, and Peter J. McNair. "Structural Brain Alterations before and after Total Knee Arthroplasty: A Longitudinal Assessment." *Pain Medicine* 19 (2018): 2166–76.

Liao, Xia, Cuiping Mao, Yuan Wang, Qingfeng Zhang, Dong-Yuan Cao, David Seminowicz, Ming Zhang, and Xiaoli Yang. "Brain Gray Matter Alterations in Chinese

Patients with Chronic Knee Osteoarthritis Pain Based on Voxel-Based Morphometry." *Medicine* (Baltimore) 97, no. 12 (March 2018): e0145.

Lin, Chia-shu. "Brain Signature of Chronic Orofacial Pain: A Systematic Review and Meta-Analysis on Neuroimaging Research of Trigeminal Neuropathic Pain and Temporomandibular Joint Disorders." *PLoS One* 9, no. 4 (2014): e94300. doi:10.1371/journal.pone.0094300.

Lipton, Richard B., Marcelo Bigal, Merle Diamond, Frederick Freitag, Michael L. Reed, and Walter Stewart. "Migraine Prevalence, Disease Burden, and the Need for Preventive Therapy." *Neurology* 68 (2007): 343–49.

Littlejohn, Geoff O. "Key Issues in Repetitive Strain Injury." In *Fibromyalgia, Chronic Fatigue Syndrome and Repetitive Strain Injury*, edited by A. Chalmers, G. O. Littlejohn, I. Strait, and F. Wolfe, 25–33. New York: Hayworth Medical Press, 1995.

Lo, Grace H., Usoh E. Ikpeama, Jeffrey B. Driban, Andrea M. Kriska, Timothy E. McAlindon, Nancy J. Petersen, Kristi L. Storti, Charles B. Eaton, Marc C. Hochberg, Rebecca D. Jackson et al. "Evidence That Swimming May Be Protective of Knee Osteoarthritis: Data from the Osteoarthritis Initiative." *Physical Medicine & Rehabilitation*, October 19, 2019. doi:10.1002/pmrj.12267.

Lo, Grace H., Sarra M. Musa, Jeffrey B. Driban, Andrea M. Kriska, Timothy E. McAlindon, Richard B. Souza, Nancy J. Petersen, Kristi Storti, Charles Eaton, Marc C. Hochberg et al. "Running Does Not Increase Symptoms or Structural Progression in People with Knee Osteoarthritis: Data from the Osteoarthritis Initiative." *Clinical Rheumatology* 37 (2018): 2497–504.

Loggia, Marco L., and Robert R. Edwards. "Brain Structural Alterations in Chronic Knee Osteoarthritis: What Can Treatment Effects Teach Us?" *Pain Medicine* 19 (2018): 2099–2100.

Lopez-Sola, Marina, Woo Choong-Wan, Jesus Pujol, Joan Deus, Ben J. Harrison, Jordi Monfort, and Tor D. Wager. "Towards a Neurophysiological Signature for Fibromyalgia." *Pain* 158 (2017): 34–47.

Luiggi-Hernandez, José G., Jean Woo, Megan Hamm, Carol M. Greco, Debra K. Weiner, and Natalia E. Morone. "Mindfulness for Chronic Low Back Pain: A Qualitative Analysis." *Pain Medicine* 19 (2018): 2138–45.

Lumley, Mark, Howard Schubiner, Nancy Lockhart, Kelley Kidwell, Steven Harte, Daniel Clauw, and David Williams. "Emotional Awareness and Expression Therapy, Cognitive Behavioral Therapy, and Education for Fibromyalgia: A Cluster-Randomized Controlled Trial." *Pain* 158 (2017): 2354–63.

MacGregor, Anne E., Jason D. Rosenberg, and Tobias Kurth. "Sex-Related Differences in Epidemiological and Clinic-Based Headache Studies." *Headache: The Journal of Head and Face Pain* 51 (2011): 843–59.

Martin, Vincent T., and Brinder Vij. "Diet and Headache: Part 1." *Headache* 56, no. 9 (October 2016): 1543–52.

Martinez-Lavin, Manuel, Mary-Carmen Amigo, Javier Coindreau, and Juan Canoso. "Fibromyalgia in Frida Kahlo's Life and Art." *Arthritis Rheumatology* 43 (2000): 708–9.

Matthias, Marianne S., and Matthew J. Bair. "The Patient–Provider Relationship in Chronic Pain Management: Where Do We Go from Here?" *Pain Medicine* 11 (2010): 1747–49.

McBeth, John, Alan J. Silman, A. Gupta, Y. H. Chiu, David Ray, Richard Moriss, Chris Dickens, and Gary J. Macfarlane. "Moderation of Psychosocial Risk Factors through Dysfunction of the Hypothalamic-Pituitary-Adrenal Stress Axis in the Onset of Chronic Widespread Musculoskeletal Pain: Findings of a Population-Based Prospective Cohort Study." *Arthritis Rheumatology* 56 (2007): 360–71.

McBeth, John, Ross Wilkie, John Bedson, Carolyn Chew-Graham, and Rosie J. Lacey. "Sleep Disturbances and Chronic Widespread Pain." *Current Rheumatology Reports* 17 (2015): 469–86.

McCrae, Christina, Jennifer M. Mundt, Ashley F. Curtis, Jason G. Craggs, and Andrew M. O'Shea. "Gray Matter Changes Following Cognitive Behavioral Therapy for Patients with Comorbid Fibromyalgia and Insomnia: A Pilot Study." *Journal of Clinical and Sleep Medicine* 14 (2018): 1595–603.

McKernan, Lindsey C., Matthew C. Lenert, Leslie J. Crofford, and Colin G. Walsh. "Outpatient Engagement and Predicted Risk of Suicide Attempts in Fibromyalgia." *Arthritis Care & Research* 71 (2019): 1255–63.

McLawhorn, Alexander S., Ashley E. Levack, Yuo-yu Lee, Yila Ge, Huong Do, and Emily R. Dodwell. "Bariatric Surgery Improves Outcomes after Lower Extremity Arthroplasty in the Morbidly Obese." *Journal of Arthroplasty* 33 (2018): 2062–69.

McLellan, Faith. "'Like Hunger, Like Thirst': Patients, Journals, and the Internet." *Lancet* 352 Supplement 2 (1999): 39–43.

Mehta, Swati, Vanessa A. Peynenburg, and Heather D. Hadjistavropoulos. "Internet-Delivered Cognitive Behaviour Therapy for Chronic Health Conditions: A Systematic Review and Meta-Analysis." *Journal of Behavioral Medicine* 42 (2019): 169–87.

Meiera, Madeline H., Avshalom Caspia, Antony Amblere, HonaLee Harrington, Renate Houts, Richard S. E. Keefe, Kay McDonald, Aimee Ward, Richie Poulton, and Terrie E. Moffitt. "Persistent Cannabis Users Show Neuropsychological Decline from Childhood to Midlife." *Proceedings of National Academy of Sciences of the United States of America* 109 (2012): E2657–64.

Meng, Xian-Guo, and Shou-Wei Yue. "Efficacy of Aerobic Exercise for Treatment of Chronic Low Back Pain: A Meta-Analysis." *American Journal of Physical Medicine & Rehabilitation* 94 (2015): 358–65.

Mezei, Lina, and Beth B. Murinson. "Pain Education in North American Medical Schools." *Journal of Pain* 12 (2011): 1199–208.

Miles, Sarah E. E., Karen P. Nicholson, and Blair H. Smith. "Chronic Pain: A Review of Its Epidemiology and Associated Factors in Population-Based Studies." *British Journal of Anaesthesia* 123 (2019): e273–83.

Moldofsky, Harvey, Phillip Scarisbrick, Richard England, and Hugh Smythe. "Musculoskeletal Symptoms and Non-REM Sleep Disturbance in Patients with 'Fibrositis Syndrome' and Healthy Subjects." *Psychosomatic Medicine* 37 (1975): 341–51.

Monaco, Annalisa, Ruggero Cattaneo, Maria Chiara Marci, Davide Pietropaoli, and Eleonora Ortu. "Central Sensitization-Based Classification for Temporomandibular Disorders: A Pathogenetic Hypothesis." *Pain Research and Management* 5 (2017): 1–13. doi:10.1155/2017/5957076.

Mucke, Martin, Tudor Phillips, Lukas Radbruch, Frank Petzke, and Winfred Hauser. "Cannabis-Based Medicines for Chronic Neuropathic Pain in Adults." *Cochrane Database of Systematic Reviews*, March 7, 2018. doi:10.1002/14651858.CD012182.

Mundal, Ingunn, Rolf Gråwe, Johan Bjørngaard, Olav Linaker, and Egil Fors. "Psychosocial Factors and Risk of Chronic Widespread Pain: An 11-Year Follow-Up Study—The HUNT Study." *Pain* 155 (2014): 1555–61.

Murray, Caitlin, Cornelius Groenewald, Rocio de Vega, and Tonya Palermo. "Long-Term Impact of Adolescent Chronic Pain on Young Adult Educational, Vocational, and Social Outcomes." *Pain* (October 21, 2019). doi:10.1097/j.pain.0000000000001732.

Nahin, Richard L., Robin Boineau, Partap S. Khalsa, Barbara J. Stussman, and Wendy J. Weber. "Evidence-Based Evaluation of Complementary Health Approaches for Pain Management in the United States." *Mayo Clinic Proceedings* 91 (2016) 91: 1292–306.

Richard L. Nahin, Barbara J. Stussman, and Patricia M. Herman. "Out of Pocket Expenditures on Complementary Health Approaches Associated with Painful Health Conditions in a Nationally Representative Adult Sample." *Journal of Pain* 15 (2015): 362–72.

Nordeman, Lena, Ronny Gunnarsson, and Kaisa Mannerkorpi. "Prevalence and Characteristics of Widespread Pain in Female Primary Health Care Patients with Chronic Low Back Pain." *Clinical Journal of Pain* 28 (2012): 65–72.

Ohayon, Maurice M., and Alan F. Schatzberg. "Chronic Pain and Major Depressive Disorder in the General Population." *Journal of Psychiatric Research* 44 (2010): 454–61.

Okifuji, Akiko, and Bradford D. Hare. "The Association between Chronic Pain and Obesity." *Journal of Pain Research* 8 (2015): 399–408.

Packiasabapathy, Senthil, and Senthilkumar Sadhasivam. "Gender, Genetics, and Analgesia: Understanding the Differences in Response to Pain Relief." *Journal of Pain Research* 11 (2018): 2729–39.

Peterlin, Lee B., Saurabh Gupta, Thomas N. Ward, and Anne MacGregor. "Sex Matters: Evaluating Sex and Gender in Migraine and Headache Research." *Headache: The Journal of Head and Face Pain* 51 (2011): 839–42.

Pietrobon, Daniela, and Michael A. Moskowitz. "Chaos and Commotion in the Wake of Cortical Spreading Depression and Spreading Depolarizations." *Nature Reviews Neuroscience* 15 (2014): 379–93.

Podoll, Klaus, and Derek Robinson. "Lewis Carroll's Migraine Experiences." *Lancet* 353 (1999): 1366.

Price, Donald D., Damien G. Finniss, and Fabrizio Benedetti. "A Comprehensive Review of the Placebo Effect: Recent Advances and Current Thought." *Annual Review of Psychology* 59 (2008): 565–90.

Probyn, Katrin, Hannah Bowers, Fiona Caldwell, Dipesh Mistry, Martin Underwood, Manjit Matharu, Tamar Pincus, and CHESS team. "Prognostic Factors for Chronic Headache: A Systematic Review." *Neurology* 89 (2017): 291–301.

Rabin, Roni Caryn. "New York Sues Family Members and Drug Distributors." *New York Times*, March 28, 2019.

Racine, Melanie. "Chronic Pain and Suicide Risk: A Comprehensive Review." *Progress in Neuro-Psychopharmacology and Biological Psychiatry* 87 (2018): 269–80.

Rathbun, Alan M., Elizabeth A. Stuart, Michelle Shardell, Michelle S. Yau, Mona Baumgarten, and Marc C. Hochberg. "Dynamic Effects of Depressive Symptoms on Osteoarthritis Knee Pain." *Arthritis Care & Research* 70 (2018): 80–88.

Reisine, Susan, Judith Fifield, Stephen Walsh, and Deborah Dauser Forrest. "Employment and Health Status Changes among Women with Fibromyalgia: A Five-Year Study." *Arthritis and Rheumatology* 59 (2008): 1735–41.

Reynolds, Michael D. "The Development of the Concept of Fibrositis." *Journal of History of Medical Allied Sciences* 38 (1983): 7–13.

Rhudy, Jamie L., Natalie Hellman, Casandra A Sturycz, Tyler A. Toledo, and Shreela Palit. "Modified Biofeedback (Conditioned Biofeedback) Promotes Anti-Nociception by Increasing the Nociceptive Flexion Reflex Threshold and Reducing Temporal Summation of Pain: A Controlled Trial." *Journal of Pain*, November 1, 2019. doi:10.1016/j.jpain.2019.10.006.

Robinson, James, Brian Theodore, Hilary Wilson, Peter Waldo, and Dennis Turk. "Determination of Fibromyalgia Syndrome after Whiplash Injuries: Methodologic Issues." *Pain* 152 (2011): 1311–16.

Romero-Reyes, Marcela, and James M. Uyanik. "Orofacial Pain Management: Current Perspectives." *Journal of Pain Research* 7 (2014): 99–115.

Russo, Antonio, Marcello Silvestro, Gioacchino Tedeschi, and Alessandro Tessitore. "Pathophysiology of Migraine: What Have We Learned from Functional Imaging?" *Current Neurology and Neuroscience Reports* 17 (2017): 95–107.

Rydman, Eric, Sari Ponzer, Rosa Brisson, Carin Ottosson, and Hans Pettersson-Järnbert. "Long-Term Follow-Up of Whiplash Injuries Reported to Insurance Companies: A Cohort Study on Patient-Reported Outcomes and Impact of Financial Compensation." *European Spine Journal* 27 (2018): 1255–61.

Sacks, Oliver. *Migraine*. Revised and expanded. New York: Vintage Books, 1999.

Sanborn, Josh. "Heroin Is Being Laced with a Terrifying New Substance: What to Know about Carfentanil." *Time*, September 12, 2016.

Sarrami, Pooria, Elizabeth Armstrong, Justine M. Naylor, and Ian A. Harris. "Factors Predicting Outcome in Whiplash Injury: A Systematic Meta-Review of Prognostic Factors." *Journal of Orthopaedic Traumatology* 18 (2017): 9–16.

Saxena, Rahul, Manish Gupta, Nilima Shankar, Sandhya Jain, and Arushi Saxena. "Effects of Yogic Intervention on Pain Scores and Quality of Life in Females with Chronic Pelvic Pain." *International Journal of Yoga* 10 (2017): 9–15.

Scarry, Elaine. *The Body in Pain: The Making and Unmaking of the World*. New York: Oxford University Press, 1985.

Schiffman, Eric, Richard Ohrbach, Edmond Truelove, John Look, Gary Anderson, Jean-Paul Goulet, Thomas List, Peter Svensson, Yoly Gonzalez-Stucker, Frank Lobbezoo et al. "Diagnostic Criteria for Temporomandibular Disorders (DC/TMD) for Clinical and Research Applications: Recommendations of the International RDC/TMD Consortium Network and Orofacial Pain Special Interest Group." *Journal of Oral Facial Pain Headache* 28 (2014): 6–27.

Schnitzer, Thomas, Richard Easton, Shirley Pang, Dennis J. Levinson, Glenn Pixton, Lars Viktrup, Isabelle Davignon, Mark T. Brown, Christine R. West, and Kenneth M. Verburg. "Effect of Tanezumab on Joint Pain, Physical Function, and Patient Global Assessment of Osteoarthritis among Patients with Osteoarthritis of the Hip or Knee: A Randomized Clinical Trial." *Journal of the American Medical Association* 322 (2019): 37–48.

Schrepf, Andrew, Steven E. Harte, Nicole Miller, Christine Fowler, Catherine Nay, David Alan Williams, Daniel J. Clauw, and Amy Rothberg. "Improvement in the Spatial Distribution of Pain, Somatic Symptoms, and Depression after a Weight Loss Intervention." *Journal of Pain* 18 (2017): 1542–50.

Seminowicz, David A., Marina Shpaner, Michael L. Keaser, G. Michael Krauthamer, John Mantegna, Julie A. Dumas, Paul Newhouse, Christopher G. Filippi, Francis J. Keefe, and Magdalena R. Naylor. "Cognitive-Behavioral Therapy Increases Prefrontal Cortex Gray Matter in Patients with Chronic Pain." *Journal of Pain* 14, no. 12 (December 2013): 1573–84.

Shillo, Pallai, Gordon Sloan, Marni Greig, Leanne Hunt, Dinesh Selvarajah, Jackie Elliott, Rajiv A. Gandhi, Iain D. Wilkinson, and Solomon Tesfaye. "Painful and Painless Diabetic Neuropathies: What Is the Difference?" *Current Diabetes Reports* 19 (2019): 32. https://doi.org/10.1007/s11892-019-1150-5.

Shim, H., J. Rose, S. Halle, and P. Shekane. "Complex Regional Pain Syndrome: A Narrative Review for the Practicing Clinician." *British Journal of Anaesthesia* 2 (2019): e424–33.

Sielski, Robert, Winfred Rief, and Julia Anna Glombiewski. "Efficacy of Biofeedback in Chronic Low Back Pain: A Meta-Analysis." *International Journal of Behavioral Medicine* 24 (2017): 25–41.

Silberg, William M., George D. Lundberg, and Robert A. Musacchio. "Assessing, Controlling, and Assuring the Quality of Medical Information on the Internet." *Journal of the American Medical Association* 277 (1997): 1244–45.

Silva, Ana Rita, Alexandra Bernardo, João Costa, Alexandra Cardoso, Paula Santos, Maria Fernanda de Mesquita, José Vaz Patto, Pedro Moreira, Maria Leonor Silva, and Patricia Padrão. "Dietary Interventions in Fibromyalgia: A Systematic Review." *Annals of Medicine* 51, suppl. (2019): 2–14. doi:10.1080/07853890.2018. 1564360.

Silverwood, Victoria, C. A. Chew-Graham, I. Raybould, B. Thomas, and S. Peters. "'If It's a Medical Issue I Would Have Covered It by Now': Learning about Fibromyalgia through the Hidden Curriculum: A Qualitative Study." *BMC Medical Education* 17 (2017): 160–96.

Sluka, Kathleen A., and Daniel J. Clauw. "Neurobiology of Fibromyalgia and Chronic Widespread Pain." *Neuroscience* 338 (2016): 114–29.

Smith, Blair, Egil Fors, Beatrice Korwisi, Antonia Barke, Paul Cameron, Lesley Colvin, Cara Richardson, Winfried Rief, and Rolf-Detlefet Treede. "The IASP Classification of Chronic Pain for ICD-11: Applicability in Primary Care." *Pain* 160 (2019): 83–87.

Sparks, Toni, Jennifer Kawi, Nancy Menzel, and Kris Hartley. "Implementation of Health Information Technology in Routine Care for Fibromyalgia: Pilot Study." *Pain Management Nursing* 17 (2016): 54–62.

Springer, Bryan D., K. M. Roberts, K. L. Bossi, S. M. Odum, and D. C. Voellinger. "What Are the Implications of Withholding Total Joint Arthroplasty in the Morbidly Obese?" *Bone and Joint Journal* 101-B, no. 7, Suppl. C (July 2019): 28–32. doi:10.1302/0301-620X.101B7.BJJ-2018-1465.R1.

Stewart, Walter F, Judith A. Ricci, Elsbeth Chee, David Morganstein, and Richard Lipton. "Lost Productive Time and Cost Due to Common Pain Conditions in the US Workforce." *Journal of the American Medical Association* 290 (2003): 2443–54.

Strøm, Vegard, Therese Kristine Dalsbø, Lise Lund Håheim, Ingvild Kirkehei, and Liv Merete Reinar. *Effect of Surgical Treatment for Temporomandibular Disorders.* Oslo: Norwegian Knowledge Centre for the Health Services, 2013.

Swift, Damon L., Neil M. Johannsen, Carl J. Lavie, Conrad P. Earnest, and Timothy S. Church. "The Role of Exercise and Physical Activity in Weight Loss and Maintenance." *Progress in Cardiovascular Diseases* 56 (2014): 441–47.

Talley, Daniel Britt. *Migraine.* Bloomington, IN: AuthorHouse, 2010.

Thomas, Katie, and Tiffany Hsu. "Johnson & Johnson's Brand Falters over Its Role in the Opioid Crisis." *New York Times,* August 27, 2019.

Thomas, Lewis. *The Medusa and the Snail.* New York: Viking Press, 1979.

Tumin, Dmitry, Adrianne Frech, Jamie L. Lynch, Vidya T. Raman, Tarun Bhalla, and Joseph D. Tobias. "Weight Gain Trajectory and Pain Interference in Young Adulthood: Evidence from a Longitudinal Birth Cohort Study." *Pain Medicine,* August 6, 2019. doi:10.1093/pm/pnz184.

Tweyman, Stanley. *René Descartes: Meditations on First Philosophy in Focus.* New York: Routledge, 1993.

Urits, Ivan, Matthew Borchart, Morgan Hasegawa, Justin Kochanski, Vwaire Orhurhu, and Omar Viswanath. "An Update of Current Cannabis-Based Pharmaceuticals in Pain Medicine." *Pain Therapy* 8 (2019): 41–51.

Urits, Ivan, Ashley Hubble, Emily Peterson, Vwaire Orhurhu, Carly A. Ernst, Alan D. Kaye, and Omar Viswanath. "An Update on Cognitive Therapy for the Management of Chronic Pain: A Comprehensive Review." *Current Pain and Headache Report* 23, no. 8 (July 10, 2019): 57.

Van Zee, Art. "The Promotion and Marketing of OxyContin: Commercial Triumph, Public Health Tragedy." *American Journal of Public Health* 99 (2009): 221–27.

Vance, Carol G. T., Ruth L. Chimenti, Dana L. Dailey, Katherine Hadlandsmyth, M. Bridget Zimmerman, Katharine Geasland, Jonathan Williams, Ericka Merriwether, Li Alemo Munters, Barbara A. Rakel et al. "Development of a Method to Maximize the Transcutaneous Electrical Nerve Stimulation Intensity in Women with Fibromyalgia." *Journal of Pain Research* 11 (2018): 2269–78.

VanDenKerkhof, Elizabeth G., Helen M. Macdonald, Gareth T. Jones, Chris Power, and Gary J. Macfarlane. "Diet, Lifestyle and Chronic Widespread Pain: Results from the 1958 British Birth Cohort Study." *Pain Research and Management* 16 (2011): 87–92.

Varinen, Aleksi, Elise Kosunen, Kari Mattila, Tuomas Koskela, and Markku Sumanen. "The Relationship between Childhood Adversities and Fibromyalgia in the General Population." *Journal of Psychosomatic Research* 99 (2017): 137–42.

Vickers, Andrew J., and Klaus Linde. "Acupuncture for Chronic Pain." *Journal of the American Medical Association* 311 (2014): 955–56.

Villareal, Dennis T., Lina Aguirre, A. Burke Gurney, Debra L. Waters, David R. Sinacore, Elizabeth Colombo, Reina Armamento-Villareal, and Clifford Qualls. "Aerobic or Resistance Exercise, or Both, in Dieting Obese Older Adults." *New England Journal of Medicine* 376 (2017): 1943–55.

Vina, Ernest, and C. Kwoh. "Epidemiology of Osteoarthritis: Literature Update." *Current Opinion in Rheumatology* 30 (2018): 160–67.

Violet, Tabetha K. "Constructing the Gendered Risk of Illness in Lyrica Ads for Fibromyalgia: Fear of Isolation as a Motivating Narrative for Consumer Demand." *Journal of Medical Humanities.* https://doi.org/10.1007/s10912-019-09575-9.

Volkow, Nora D., and A. Thomas McLellan. "Opioid Abuse in Chronic Pain: Misconceptions and Mitigation Strategies." *New England Journal of Medicine* 374 (2016): 1253–63.

Vučković, Sonja, Dragana Srebro, Katarina Savić Vujović, Čedomir Vučetić, and Milica Prostran. "Cannabinoids and Pain: New Insights from Old Molecules." *Frontiers in Pharmacology* 9 (November 13, 2018): 1259. doi:10.3389/fphar.2018.01259.

Wager, Tor D., Lauren Y. Atlas, Martin A. Lindquist, Mathieu Roy, Choong-Wan Woo, and Ethan Kross. "An fMRI-Based Neurologic Signature of Physical Pain." *New England Journal of Medicine* 368 (2013): 1388–97.

Wang, Chenchen, Christopher H. Schmid, Roger A. Fielding, William F. Harvey, Kieran Reid, Lori Lyn Price, Jeffrey B. Driban, Robert A. Kalish, Ramel Rones, and Timothy McAlindon. "Effect of Tai Chi versus Aerobic Exercise for Fibromyalgia: Comparative Effectiveness Randomized Controlled Trial." *British Medical Journal* 360 (2018): k851. doi:10.1136/bmj.k851.

Wang, Chenchen, Christopher H. Schmid, Ramel Rones, Robert Kalish, Janeth Yinh, Don L. Goldenberg, Yoojin Lee, and Timothy McAlindon. "A Randomized Trial of Tai Chi for Fibromyalgia." *New England Journal of Medicine* 363 (2010): 743–54.

Wang, Claudia, Kaigang Li, Arkopal Choudhury, and Susan Gaylord. "Trends in Yoga, Tai Chi, and Qigong Use among US Adults, 2002–2017." *American Journal of Public Health* 109 (2019): 755–61.

Warren, John W., Patricia Langenberg, and Daniel J Clauw. "The Number of Existing Functional Somatic Syndromes (FSSs) Is an Important Risk Factor for New, Different FSSs." *Journal of Psychosomatic Research* 74, no. 1 (2013): 12–17.

Whitlock, Elizabeth L., L. Grisell Diaz-Ramirez, M. Maria Glymour, W. John Bosardin, Kenneth E. Covinsky, and Alexander K. Smith. "Association between Persistent Pain and Memory Decline and Dementia in a Longitudinal Cohort of Elders." *Journal of the American Medical Association Internal Medicine* 177 (2017): 1146–53.

Wolfe, Frederick, Hugh A. Smythe, Muhammed B. Yunus, Robert M. Bennett, Claire Bombardier, Don L. Goldenberg, Peter Tugwell, S. M. Campbell, Micha Abeles, and Patricia Clark. "The American College of Rheumatology 1990 Criteria for the Classification of Fibromyalgia." *Arthritis Rheumatology* 33 (1990): 160–72.

Woodworth, Davis C., Adelle Dagher, Adam Curatolo, Monisha Sachdev, Cody Ashe-McNalley, Bruce D. Naliboff, Jennifer Labus, J. Richard Landis, Jason J. Kutch, Emeran A. Mayer et al., "Changes in Brain White Matter Structure Are Associated with Urine Proteins in Urologic Chronic Pelvic Pain Syndrome (UCPPS): A MAPP Network Study." *PLos One* 13, no. 12 (December 5, 2018): e0206807. doi:10.1371/journal.pone.0206807.

Woolf, Virginia. "On Being Ill." In *The Criterion*, by T. S. Eliot. London: Hogarth Press, 1926.

Wu, Yin, Blair T. Johnson, Rebecca L. Acabchuk, Shiqi Chen, Holly K. Lewis, Jill Livingston, Crystal L. Park, and Linda S. Pescatello. "Yoga as Antihypertensive Lifestyle Therapy: A Systematic Review and Meta-Analysis." *Mayo Clinic Proceedings* 94 (2019): 432–46.

Xin-chang, Zhang, Hao Chen, Wen-tao Xu, Yang-yang Song, Ya-hui Gu, and Guang-xia Ni. "Acupuncture Therapy for Fibromyalgia: A Systematic Review and Meta-Analysis of Randomized Controlled Trials." *Journal of Pain Research* 12 (2019): 527–42.

Yanes, Julio A. "Toward a Multimodal Framework of Brainstem Pain-Modulation Circuits in Migraine." *Journal of Neuroscience* 39 (2019): 6035–37.

Yu, Angus, Bjorn Tam, Christopher Lai, Doris S. F. Yu, Jean Woo, Ka-Fai Chung, Stanley Hui, Justina Y. Liu, Gao X. Wei, and Parco Siu. "Revealing the Neural Mechanisms Underlying the Beneficial Effects of Tai Chi: A Neuroimaging Perspective." *American Journal of Chinese Medicine* 46 (2018): 231–59.

Zeidan, Fadel, Katherine T. Martucci, Robert A. Kraft, Nakia S. Gordon, John G. McHaffie, and Robert C. Coghill. "Brain Mechanisms Supporting the Modulation of Pain by Mindfulness Meditation." *Journal of Neuroscience* 31 (2011): 5540–48.

Zeng, Chao, Maureen Dubreuil, Marc R. LaRochelle, Na Lu, Jie Wei, Hyon K. Choi, Guanghua Lei, and Yuqing Zhang. "Association of Tramadol with All-Cause Mortality among Patients with Osteoarthritis." *Journal of the American Medical Association* 321 (2019): 969–82.

Zhao, Sizheng Steven, Stephen J. Duffield, and Nicola J. Goodson. "The Prevalence and Impact of Comorbid Fibromyalgia in Inflammatory Arthritis." *Best Practice & Research Clinical Rheumatology* 33, no. 3 (June 2019): 101423. doi:10.1016/j.berh.2019.06.005.

Zilliox, Lindsay. "Neuropathic Pain: Selected Topics in Outpatient Neurology." *CONTINUUM: Lifelong Learning in Neurology* 23, no. 2 (2017): 512–32. doi:10.1212/CON.0000000000000462.

Zorina-Lichtenwalter, Katerina, Carolina Beraldo Meloto, Samar Khoury, and Luda Diatchenko. "Genetic Predictors of Human Chronic Pain Conditions." *Neuroscience* 338 (2016): 36–62.

INDEX

ABOUT THE AUTHOR

Dr. Don Goldenberg is emeritus professor of medicine, Tufts University School of Medicine, and a member of the adjunct faculty, departments of medicine and nursing, at Oregon Health Sciences University, in Portland, Oregon, where he resides. Dr. Goldenberg has published more than two hundred articles in scientific journals covering many areas of arthritis, rheumatology and chronic pain. His book, *Fibromyalgia: A Leading Expert's Guide to Understanding and Getting Relief from the Pain That Won't Go Away* (2002), sold more than twenty thousand copies in the United States and the United Kingdom. He received the Marion Ropes Lifetime Achievement Award from the Massachusetts Arthritis Foundation in 2008 and was named a Master of the American College of Rheumatology in 2009. He is the section editor for the section on pain disorders in rheumatology on the UpToDate website, https://www.uptodate.com/home. Dr. Goldenberg has been included in each edition of *The Best Doctors in America* and selected as one of the "Best Doctors in Boston" by *Boston* magazine. His medical expertise has made him widely sought out for commentary on national and local television. He's been interviewed on *Today* and *Good Morning America*, and his work on chronic illnesses has been covered in the *New York Times*, the *Boston Globe*, and the *New Yorker*.